He who dwells in the shelter
of the Most High will abide in
the shadow of the Almighty.
        I will say to the LORD,
"My refuge and my fortress,
  my God, in whom I trust."
        For He will command
His angels concerning you to
guard you in all your ways.

Psalm 91:1–2

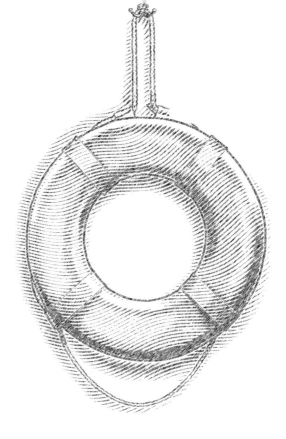

Blessings & Prayers

FOR THOSE WITH CANCER

A Devotional Companion

By Karen Boerger and Annetta Dellinger

CONCORDIA PUBLISHING HOUSE · SAINT LOUIS

Compiled and written by Karen Boerger and Annetta Dellinger

Unless otherwise indicated, Scripture quotations from the ESV Bible® (The Holy Bible, English Standard Version®), copyright © 2001 by Crossway Bibles, a publishing ministry of Good News Publishers. Used by permission. All rights reserved.

Scripture quotations marked NIV are taken from the Holy Bible, New International Version®. NIV®. Copyright © 1973, 1978, 1984 by Biblica, Inc.™ Used by permission of Zondervan. All rights reserved.

Hymn texts and prayers marked LSB are from *Lutheran Service Book*, copyright © 2006 Concordia Publishing House. All rights reserved.

The catechism quotations are from *Luther's Small Catechism with Explanation*, copyright © 1986, 1991 Concordia Publishing House. All rights reserved.

Prayers marked *Portals of Prayer* are adapted from *Portals of Prayer*, January–March 2010, copyright © 2009 Concordia Publishing House. All rights reserved.

Prayers marked *Visitation* are adapted from *Visitation: Resources for the Care of Souls* by Arthur A. Just and Scot A. Kinnaman, copyright © 2008 Concordia Publishing House. All rights reserved.

Prayers marked *Blessings* are adapted from *Blessings and Prayers for Caregivers* by Annetta Dellinger and Karen Boerger, copyright © 2010 Concordia Publishing House. All rights reserved.

Manufactured in the United States of America

Library of Congress Cataloging-in-Publication Data

Boerger, Karen.
  Blessings and prayers for those with cancer : a devotional companion / by Karen Boerger and Annetta Dellinger.
    p. cm.
  ISBN 978-0-7586-2672-1
  1. Cancer--Patients--Prayers and devotions. I. Dellinger, Annetta E. II. Title.

BV4910.33.B64 2011
242'.4--dc22
                                                    2011013508

1 2 3 4 5 6 7 8 9 10   20 19 18 17 16 15 14 13 12 11

*This book is dedicated to special friends
who have walked the cancer journey
and helped us with this book.*

*Thank you, Ann, Lyla, Marti,
Millie, and Ruth.*

We love you!

Table of Contents

Preface

Cancer survivors have strengths that amaze everyone.

They bear hardships, and they carry burdens.

They smile when they want to scream;
    they sing when they want to cry.

They cry when they're happy
    and laugh when they're nervous.

They fight for what they believe in.

They don't take no for an answer when they believe there's a better solution.

They research and then research some more.

They look forward because they trust in the Lord.

They bear the indignities of cancer with patience.

They go to the doctor with a frightened friend.

They cry when their children excel
    and cheer when their friends succeed.

They are happy when they hear about a birth or a wedding.

They grieve when a cancer buddy dies.

They pray and give thanks for the close friends
who give them strength,
    and they find strength when they think
        they have none left.
They know that a hug and a kiss can send a
heart soaring.
They drive to, fly to, walk to, run to, phone, or
e-mail another cancer victim to show how much
they care.
They keep things going because they have heart.
They bring joy, hope, love, compassion,
and ideas.
They give spiritual support to their family
and friends.
They nurture their children with the love shown
in the gift of a Savior.
They pray without ceasing.

We acknowledge the gifts of cancer survivors,
    and we remember those who suffer no
        more and walk in newness of life.

Karen and Annetta

Meditations

Love
Why Save the Chemo Wig?

> *Faith is the assurance of things hoped for, the
> conviction of things not seen.* Hebrews 11:1

On a sunny spring day, Jan decided to tackle the bedroom closet. With closet space at a premium in her small apartment, it was time to organize summer clothes and pack winter items away. As she surveyed the task at hand, Jan looked up to the top shelf and saw her wig. As she took it down, she thought, *Why am I keeping this? I should just toss it.*

Holding the wig, Jan thought back to five years ago when chemotherapy ruled her life. Losing her hair wasn't a pleasant experience, but having the wig helped her remain stable to meet the world head-on. The scarves she wore when she didn't want to don the wig were repurposed, now adding color to her day wear. But why save the chemo wig?

Perhaps Jan's wig serves as a badge of courage. Perhaps it still sits in her closet as a functional wig, waiting just in case it's needed once more. Perhaps now it says to her, "I'm okay." It made her feel beautiful at a time when she didn't feel that way. It covered her when she felt exposed. Perhaps Jan's wig in the closet is a combination of all three.

Many emotions run through the minds of cancer survivors. For them, the disease never really goes away; it just gets put aside. As Jan unconsciously hugged her wig to her heart, she was reminded of God's faithfulness.

Jan has a great faith in God and in His power in her life. She trusts Him more than anything else. And during chemo, when she was at her lowest point physically, Jan's faith had never been stronger. As she thought back to that time and to the peace from God that she felt, she bowed her head and prayed, "Dear Father, You are the love of my life. You have been with me every moment, through the good and the bad. You are my all in all. I do not fear the future because I know You are with me. And I know that whatever happens in this life, You will take me through it to the better life ahead. For Jesus' sake. Thank You, Father! Amen."

Love

A Dog Named Lucky

For God so loved the world, that He gave
His only Son, that whoever believes in Him
should not perish but have eternal life. John 3:16

Lucky was a special dog, a loving and funny character who had a special place in Mary and Jim's family. With big brown eyes and long soft ears, Lucky was the cutest thief you'd ever want to meet. When Mary and Jim had overnight guests, they warned their friends not to leave their luggage open because Lucky would help himself to whatever struck his fancy. Inevitably, someone would forget, and then something would come up missing. Mary or Jim would go to Lucky's toy box in the basement, and there the treasure would be, nestled among Lucky's favorite toys. Lucky always stashed his finds in his toy box and was very particular that *his toys stayed* in the box.

It happened that Mary found out she had breast cancer. She believed she was going to die of this disease; she was sure it was fatal.

Mary scheduled the double mastectomy, fear riding her shoulders. The night before she was to go to the hospital, she cuddled with Lucky. A thought struck her—*what would happen to Lucky?* Although the three-year-old dog liked Jim, he was Mary's dog through and through. *If I die, Lucky will be devastated,* Mary thought. *He won't understand that I didn't want to leave him.* The thought made her sadder than thinking of her own death.

The double mastectomy was harder on Mary than her doctors had anticipated, and she was hospitalized for more than two weeks. Jim faithfully took Lucky for his evening walks, but the dog drooped and whined and was miserable. Finally, the day came for Mary to leave the hospital. When she arrived home, she was so exhausted that she couldn't even make it up the steps to her bedroom. Jim made his wife as comfortable as he could on the couch and left the house to run some quick errands. Lucky stood watching Mary, but he didn't come to her when she called. It made Mary sad, but fatigue soon overcame her and she dozed.

When Mary woke from her nap, she knew something was wrong. She couldn't move her head, and her body felt heavy and hot. Panic soon gave way to laughter, though, when Mary realized the problem. She was covered, literally blanketed, in every treasure Lucky owned!

While she slept, the sorrowing dog made trip after trip to the basement and back, bringing his beloved mistress his favorite things in life. He had covered her with his love.

Mary forgot about dying. Instead, she and Lucky began living again. As the days went on and Mary began to heal, she and Lucky began taking walks together. Short distances at first and then walking farther and farther every day.

It's been twelve years since Mary's surgery, and she is still cancer-free. Lucky? He still steals treasures and stashes them in his toy box, but Mary remains his greatest treasure.
—Author Unknown

This story has circulated on the Internet for years, but its message of devotion and love remain compelling. It is reminiscent of the love Jesus shows us. He covered us with His saving love when He laid down His life on the cross. As the hymnwriter says, "What wondrous love is this!" We can rest assured that through the death and resurrection of Jesus, we are God's treasures. Jesus took our sins upon Himself and blanketed us with forgiving love. What wondrous love, indeed!

Acts of Kindness
Jesus Loves You, Mommy!

> God is our refuge and strength, a very present
> help in trouble. Psalm 46:1

Angie enjoys helping her daughter, Alicia, at her lemonade stand. Together they make lemonade and package homemade cookies in bags to sell for a quarter apiece. Angie often comments that her daughter was so young to have been through so much, but she adds that Alicia was made stronger by all of it. Now, Angie gladly helps Alicia share her kindness and raise quarters for cancer research.

During her chemo treatments, when Angie was so weak she could barely lift her head, Alicia was her little helper. Bringing a cold compress for her head helped keep the "queasies" at bay. Alicia's little hand, so soft and warm, patting her mommy as she sat on the side of the bed put a smile on Angie's face and made her remember what she was fighting for. Every night, Alicia came to Angie's bedroom and sang "Jesus Loves Me" before going to bed. After her prayers and song, Alicia would whisper, "Jesus loves you, Mommy, and so do I."

It's the little things, the intentional acts of kindness, that will long be remembered. After five years of being cancer-free, the bladder cancer seems a distant season in Angie's life, yet she can vividly recall special touches of love—cards so funny she laughed every time she read them, honeysuckle lotion that remains her favorite to this day, a neighbor going to the grocery store for them and each time bringing back treats tied with a bow.

God's act of kindness was also intentional as He gave us a Savior so that all who believe are assured of living with Him eternally. God had a plan to reconcile His children by heaping our sins upon His only Son, Jesus. Jesus intentionally took our sins upon Himself and suffered a painful death so that all believers are healed by His blood. God is our strength. In these not-so-little acts, we find refuge in all the days of our trouble. His Word and Sacraments—ultimate kindnesses—renew us with God's forgiveness and, in turn, give us strength. May we always remember that Jesus loves us!

Attitude
Three Hairs—A New Attitude

A joyful heart is good medicine, but a crushed spirit dries up the bones. Proverbs 17:22

The following story has appeared many times on the Internet, but it's a favorite of many and bears repeating:

There once was a woman who woke up one morning, looked in the mirror, and saw that she had only three hairs on her head. "Well," she said, "I think I'll braid my hair today." So she did, and she had a wonderful day.

The next day, this same woman woke up, looked in the mirror, and saw that she had only two hairs on her head. "Hmm," she said, "today I'm going to wear my hair in pigtails." So she did, and she had a fun, fun day.

The next day, she woke up, looked in the mirror, and noticed that there was only one hair on her head. "Today," she exclaimed, "I will wear my pair in a ponytail!" So she did, and she had another great day.

The next day, she woke up and saw that she had no hair on her head. "Great! Today I don't have to fix my hair!"

If only all of us shared this attitude—to see the blessings and not the burdens of whatever situation we're in. Satan knows that our lack of contentment can lead to a poor attitude and, ultimately, loss of faith. He will attack our weaknesses and fears at every turn. He'll use anything to shake our faith in our amazing God.

In Matthew 6:25–34, Jesus tells us not to worry, that the Father gives us what we need. He shows us the flowers of the field and the birds of the air as proof. And He reminds us that the joy of our hearts is knowing God loves us so much that He gave His "only Son, that whoever believes in Him should not perish but have eternal life" (John 3:16).

Now, isn't that a great attitude?

Hope
The Power of Second Opinions

The prayer of a righteous person has great power as it is working. James 5:16

John was shocked to learn that he had prostate cancer. There was no family history that suggested he should be concerned about cancer. He was active, had no symptoms, and always ate nutritious foods. But when he was diagnosed, he became an "encyclopedia of knowledge" about prostate cancer. This was one way he could wage war against cancer.

His battle began with an annual physical that included a Prostate-Specific Antigen (PSA) blood test. His doctor found no irregularities in the physical exam, and he had a fairly normal PSA level. However, that level had risen during the previous two years, and this caught the doctor's attention. (A rise of .75 percent or more per year can be an indicator that cancer is present.)

John was sent to a urologist for a biopsy; however, he decided to have a less-invasive test (FPSA) done to measure the percentage of free versus bound PSA. His result was 13 percent. (Anything under 20 percent is an indicator of cancer.) John had a second FPSA test done, and it came back with the same 13 percent. He had confirmation.

John decided then to go forward with the biopsy. When the lab report came back, it was negative for cancer. John said, "I was happy, but I was still skeptical because the other two tests warned that something was wrong."

So John sought another opinion. The slides of the ten samples taken during his biopsy were sent to a major cancer hospital, and the original lab assured John they would reexamine the samples as well. One week later, he received results from both labs.

John had cancer.

The good news was that his cancer was encapsulated, meaning it had not spread outside the prostate gland. The bad news was the possibility of impotence, incontinence, and other symptoms of the aftermath of the surgery.

Now, ten years after his diagnosis, treatment, and recovery, John volunteers at the same cancer hospital where he was treated. He stresses the importance of testing and retesting to ensure complete accuracy. John says, "My faith in God grew stronger almost daily. I prayed several times a day. It was like a continuous dialogue—just God and I, discussing my fears and concerns. Here it is ten years later, and I still talk with God as much as I did then. It was a good habit to develop, and it brings such peace to my life. God has been my comfort and guide every step of the way. It doesn't get much better than that."

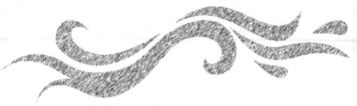

Friendship
What a Blessing You Are, My Friend!

A friend loves at all times. Proverbs 17:17

After Shelley was diagnosed with bone cancer, she prayed, "What's wrong, God? What are You telling me?" She was so overwhelmed with the diagnosis that she had to work doubly hard so she wasn't distracted from her day-to-day teaching schedule.

How she loved those children! For a few hours each day, she set her worry aside and became totally absorbed in their young lives. The hours outside of the classroom, however, were a different story.

One day she said, "I'm trying to keep up my students' spirits and make sure they are leading lives as normal as they can. But when the evenings and weekends roll around, my strength isn't as great as I would like it to be. The day in the classroom saps my energy. I feel like I'm failing my own children."

Shelley is a single parent, so trying to maintain the daily routine and be at all the activities of her two teenagers was challenging. Her spirit was willing, but her body was weak. Then Shelley's friend Patty came up with a way to help. Patty volunteered to take her video camera to some of the events Shelley couldn't attend. Later, Shelley could watch the video playback with her children at home and enjoy the event with them.

Months later, Shelley said, "You are such a good friend, Patty. What would I have done without you during my crisis? The videos you took at the kids' events were so precious to me. The kids and I had such fun watching them. Joshua made popcorn, and Haley poured the soda. We've watched the videos more than once, and the kids' special commentary has been precious. What a blessing you are, my friend! I love you."

When we see the amazing love Jesus has for us, we can't help but share that love with others. His arms lovingly outstretched on the cross for us move us to extend our arms in love to others. Then, when we see the needs all around us, we respond with Christ's love and compassion. As we serve others, we honor our Savior, the ultimate Servant. Because He loves us, Jesus gave His all so we might have forgiveness and live with Him eternally. Now, that's the blessing of our best Friend!

"In Him we live and move and have our being" (Acts 17:28).

Joy
The Flutist

> *Make a joyful noise to the L*ORD, *all the earth; break forth into joyous song and sing praises!* Psalm 98:4

Ruth dreaded the long time she would have to sit and watch the chemo drip into her arm. And it wasn't just the two or three hours of sitting that bothered her—it was also the days afterward when she would be weak and sick. She tried the pills to help suppress the nausea, but they didn't seem to work. To her, time was such a factor during those days. Having cancer was bad enough, but she was frustrated about wasting time with the sickness that her treatment brought on. Ruth knew that patience was not her strongest virtue.

One day as she was receiving chemo, Ruth tried to distract herself by reading a book. As she read, she began to hear beautiful music coming from somewhere nearby. She looked up and there, at the other end of the room, was a young lady, tethered to her own chemo bag, playing the flute. Ruth marveled that the flutist could play an instrument with the IV drip. It was all Ruth could do to turn pages of her book comfortably, and here was another patient putting on a live concert!

The young woman finished her chemo treatment at about the same time Ruth did, so she took an opportunity to talk with her. The young lady, Kim Liu, told Ruth that she had been with the local symphony orchestra for ten years. Her breast cancer was back for the second time, and she was trying a new chemo medicine that had no side effects so far. Kim said that she decided to use the time to practice and give joy to the other patients and the staff of the clinic. No time wasted there! She was so upbeat and positive that Ruth felt better just talking with her.

Ruth enjoyed her new friend's music so much that she looked forward to going to treatments when Kim was also there. Ruth just closed her eyes and listened to the music of the flute. She let her mind create scenes that went along with the rise and fall of the notes—sheep on a hillside with a babbling brook, a church setting, a city just awakening in the morning.

Kim's gift of music made Ruth's heart soar. Praise God for special people such as Kim who come unexpectedly into the lives of others and remind them of the beauty and joy of the moment. It's such a blessing to be so lovingly cared for by our heavenly Father!

Faith
"What Did I Do to Deserve This?"

Count it all joy, my brothers, when you meet trials of various kinds, for you know that the testing of your faith produces steadfastness. James 1:2–3

When Karen's father was diagnosed with colon cancer, the entire family was stunned. They listened to the doctor talk about the surgical solution—a colostomy. The procedure seemed drastic, but at that time there was no alternative, even when the cancer had been caught early as it was in this case.

Her father had gone to the doctor because he had pain in his upper abdomen. The doctor thought it might be caused by adhesions from previous surgeries. Later, the surgeon thought the same thing. But when the preliminary tests were complete, they revealed a small polyp in the colon that looked suspicious. Further tests verified that it was cancer. Because of the placement of the polyp, the only treatment was an irreversible colostomy.

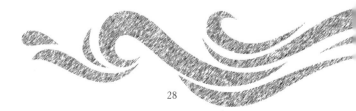

The night following the surgery, as Karen's father tried to move in his bed to find a bit of relief from the pain, Karen heard him say, "What did I do to deserve this?" He didn't realize that Karen was sitting in the room; his question was directed to his heavenly Father. But Karen had to ponder the question too. *What would God's answer be?*

She thought about what had prompted her dad to go to the doctor in the first place and about the many people who had encouraged him to consult his doctor. He had felt pain in the upper abdomen—and perhaps God allowed it to motivate him to see the doctor because cancer was found in the lower bowel. (The upper abdominal pain was not an issue after the surgery.) The Lord allows people and circumstances into our lives for a reason. We need to be open to His help and thankful for the care He gives us through others.

By faith, we believe in God, our Creator. By faith, we trust in His ultimate care through Christ Jesus, our Master Physician.

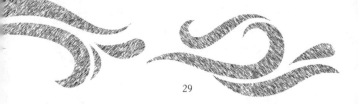

29

Help
Pass It On

For You have been my help, and in the shadow of Your wings I will sing for joy. Psalm 63:7

David was diagnosed with a brain tumor. Everyone wanted to know what they could do to help. Within a short time, his church family, school family, friends, and relatives all came together via the phone prayer tree, social media, and other avenues to coordinate caregivers and prayer partners.

Many people from across the country offered help not only with prayers, but also with food, housekeeping, and more. The ministry to David continued for months. He said, "I was so encouraged. I felt loved and cared for—not just for me, but also for my family."

After David recovered from surgery and returned to work, he was determined to help others in the same way he had been helped. He contacted the Random Acts of Kindness organization to offer his help, and he became a member of the Caring Hearts committee in his church to help with practical tasks that would benefit those in need.

What's more, his love for his Lord has become the first priority in life. Before his cancer, David often missed church services. Now, he regularly attends worship and has joined an adult Sunday School class. David said, "My tumor was a wake-up call to what is truly important in my life. I don't know what I was thinking before. I was putting other things before God, and He is the one who gave me all the blessings that I enjoy each day! My cancer slowed me down and made me think. Frankly, I'm grateful that having cancer showed me God's mercy and taught me how I can serve Him and share His love and care with others. There is nothing more important. All praise and glory to Him!"

Serving in Love
Serving by Being Served

> As each has received a gift, use it to serve one another,
> as good stewards of God's varied grace. 1 Peter 4:10

Many of us have lived our entire lives under the umbrella of Christian love. We show that love by reaching out to others, as the Good Samaritan did. "By love serve one another" has been our motto. "Christ came not to be served, but to serve" has been our example. Servanthood is the result of our Christian living. We want to give, to help, to reach out to others, finding joy and satisfaction because we do. We have learned what Paul learned and spoke to the Ephesian elders: "It is more blessed to give than to receive" (Acts 20:35).

The irony of this is that many of us feel more comfortable serving than in being served. In fact, we may even feel *uncomfortable* when we are served, uncomfortable at being the *object* of the concern of others as we battle cancer or other diseases. It is a lesson in humility that one way of serving might be to give others the opportunity to serve us.

Other people experience as much satisfaction in serving us as we do when we serve them. Not to accept their services graciously may be denying them the very opportunity for service that *they* need as much as we do. Another way to think about this is that the circle of love is completed when others serve us and we let them: their meeting our physical and spiritual needs of the moment allows us to help meet their need to be of help and service to us. Receiving care is ministry too, a ministry into which we are sometimes thrust by our own helplessness, a ministry in which we learn that there are times when it is better to receive than to give (W. J. Fields, *An Odyssey through Cancer* © 1996 Wheat Ridge Ministries, pp. 10–11). Used with permission.

Forgiveness
Betrayal

> *Bear with each other and forgive whatever*
> *grievances you may have against one another.*
> *Forgive as the Lord forgave you.*
> Colossians 3:13 NIV

June 10 Journal Entry

Dear God,
Here I am again with my journal ramblings. But today I'm writing happy thoughts. You and I both

know that it's been a long time coming. When I look back over the last three years and twelve notebooks with hundreds and hundreds of filled pages, I relive those days all over again.

The day I received the news that the radiologist who had read my March scans had been wrong was the lowest day of my "cancer life." I had been so thrilled after hearing the "good" report that the cancer had not returned. I remember the lovely candlelight dinner my husband prepared for me to celebrate this news. But a mere three months later, I learned that not only had I *not* been cancer-free, but the tumors that were there in March had grown substantially by June.

The anger I felt can only be compared to overwhelming rage, and betrayal oozed out of every fiber of my being. I felt totally consumed with resentment against this one individual who couldn't read an x-ray correctly. At the time, I couldn't see how I could ever forgive him, but Your Holy Spirit led me to Your Word time and time again.

Even when I was so weak that I couldn't hold the Bible in my hands, my husband read to me, or I listened to recordings of the Psalms. Your Word soothed my spirit and, slowly, over time, I was able to realize that the radiologist only made a mistake.

It was a big one, to be sure, but that's all it was, a mistake, and I was the only one affected by it.

I make mistakes daily in thoughts, words, and actions, but I am assured of Your forgiveness, and You always keep Your promises. If I am to acknowledge Your love and forgiveness, Lord, how can I hold bitterness in my heart?

Yes, precious Father, after being in the Word, persistently looking for Your comfort and care, I feel my heart has opened up to a new resurgence of hope. It has taken me a long time to get to this point, but I'm here, and I feel such freedom!

There is even greater freedom ahead as I look to my eternal home with You . . . freedom from pain, freedom from emotional stress, freedom from sin. I know that Jesus bought my freedom on the cross so that I may enjoy true freedom to be with You, Father. Thank You for being in my life! I love You!

Your daughter in Christ,

Hope
The Diagnosis

You are my hiding place and my shield;
I hope in Your word. Psalm 119:114

Kay remembers that the car ride home from the doctor's office was one of the quietest rides she had ever taken. Both she and her husband were in separate worlds of thought, and neither felt like talking. What was there to say? They had to grapple with their own thoughts and feelings before they knew what to say to each other.

Kay had been having pain in her left breast for a few weeks and made an appointment to see her gynecologist. Although she felt no lump, the doctor detected a slight thickening and set up an appointment for her to see a specialist.

Kay was relieved that her husband drove the hour-long trip to and from the appointment, because she wasn't sure she would have been in the right frame of mind to drive home. After giving her medical history (yes, she has many relatives who have dealt with cancer), Kay had a sonogram. She admits that at first it was interesting to watch the screen, but she was filled with dread when the doctor said, "I don't like the looks of that." He asked the nurse to prepare Kay for a needle biopsy.

As she awaited the procedure, she felt an odd combination of calm and terror. She told herself, Well, if I have to have this procedure, at least I can be glad that I didn't have to wait for another appointment and have to cope with the tension and nerves for several days.

Local anesthetic made the procedure painless; however, the grinding sound of the instrument used to take samples was nerve-jarring. And Kay's anxiety increased when the test results took longer because of a holiday weekend.

During those days, Kay benefited from a supportive family and frequent prayers to God, which kept her uplifted by reminding her of God's steadfastness. Her faith in God's promises and mercy never wavered. Despite her nervousness about the test results, she knew God would be her strength, her hope, and her constant companion.

Faith

Poodle Hair

> *For the LORD sees not as man sees: man looks on the outward appearance, but the LORD looks on the heart.* 1 Samuel 16:7

"It's vanity, I know, but I'm having a really difficult time. First I was bald, and now I have 'poodle' hair! All I lack is a little pink bow on top of my head. Aaack!"

Meeting Darla for the first time was delightful for Barb. Darla had a sharp wit, keen insight, and a joyful love for her Lord. But Darla's comment about her hair took Barb by surprise. Barb asked, "What was your hair like before chemo?"

"Light brown and straight. I don't look in the mirror very often now because it's not me. All these years I have seen and combed straight brown hair, and now the reflection in the mirror looks like it doesn't belong to me! My new hair has some of my brown color, but the salt-and-pepper look is new. I'm not allowed to color my hair yet because of my treatments. Besides that—look at all these curls! Where did they come from? I had straight hair before!"

"Some people pay a lot of money to have curls like yours," Barb said. "I think your hair looks nice."

"Thank you, Barb. But it's just so different that it's a shock. After all I've been through, and I can't even see me when I look in the mirror. It'll take me some time to get used to it, that's for sure. Did I tell you that my brother shaved his head when I was bald? That was so sweet of him."

"Wow! That was really nice of him to do that. But, you know, Darla, although many people look at the outward appearance, it's what's on the inside that truly matters. That's what you would say to someone else in the same circumstance. As Christians, we know that whether it's our hair or some other outward change, the real transformation takes place in our heart. Jesus transforms us. We have been bought and paid for by His blood, shed on the cross for each one of us. He knows us. 'The Lord knows those who are His' (2 Timothy 2:19). Our names are written in His Book of Life."

"You're right, Barb. Through the tough times of treatment, my faith grew even stronger because I clung to the Scriptures. We're so blessed to have such a loving God."

"Amen, Darla. Amen!"

Humor

The Sky Is Falling! The Sky Is Falling!

For everything there is a season, and a time
for every matter under heaven: . . . a time to weep,
and a time to laugh; a time to mourn,
and a time to dance. Ecclesiastes 3:1, 4

Isn't *Chicken Little* a charming story? It has such a good message: have courage. Just the thought of Chicken Little running around telling everyone she knows "The sky is falling!" makes us smile.

People with cancer have courage to face the unknown. When the diagnosis is made, there can be many tears shed ("a time to weep"), but there are many times to smile and laugh. Some of the following stories may make "a cheerful face" (Proverbs 15:13). Although some may not be so funny at first, consider how these individuals dealt with their situation. Then smile.

1. Scared, angry, wondering why the cancer hadn't been detected three years earlier when Marie first discovered the lump, she said to her doctor, "You can't tell me this today! I am 49 years old! You can tell me this when I'm 54, but not now!" Marie has long since wondered what possessed her to say 54. Why not 84 or 94? At her next appointment, she sincerely apologized to her doctor for that outburst. It's now twenty-four years later, and Marie praises God for His forgiveness and healing.

2. Lucy's hair really fell out one day when she was taking a shower. Reality set in when she saw her own bird's nest on the shower floor. It was not a funny sight, but the good news was that when Lucy was first diagnosed, the oncology nurse suggested that she pick out a wig right away. Lucy took that advice, so that morning, after her hair finally fell out, she simply called the shop,

picked up her wig, and took it straight to her hairdresser. The stylist trimmed it to look just like Lucy's style. After that, she often received compliments from people who had no idea she was a cancer patient. That made her smile!

3. Christine, a kindergarten teacher, was overwhelmed when one of the moms asked if she'd be able to teach. She surely wanted to, but she didn't know how six weeks of radiation would affect her. When the mom suggested that she and other moms could help in the classroom, Christine said they would need clearance from the principal and school board. The volunteer mom smiled and said, "We've already done that, and they have okayed our plan." Wow! What a boost! The volunteer moms did all her bulletin boards. A mom was in the classroom every day to assist and to insist that Christine *sit* to teach. For Christine, being on the receiving end of this kind of care was a humbling experience and a tremendous gift, because it meant that throughout her treatment she could remain in the classroom with the children she loved so much.

4. Someone asked Carolyn to describe what chemotherapy was like. She told them, "It was like having Clorox in my stomach. But I simply accepted the sick feeling for a day or two and knew it would improve. Chicken noodle soup and I became close associates!"

5. Talking with God daily, even hourly, is a common practice for those with cancer or those who have gone through extensive treatments. For example, during his battle with cancer, Mark prayed constantly. As he did, his relationship with his Lord grew even stronger as he learned what it meant to fully rely on Him. Mark prayed for complete recovery. But if that wasn't God's plan, he asked that God would walk with him through whatever was ahead, and that He would increase the faith of his entire family. Mark prayed for the Holy Spirit to reign in his heart and show him how and where he could serve God. Then, sense of humor intact, Mark asked God to paint that door red so he wouldn't miss it.

In all of life's challenges, there is a time to weep and a time to laugh. Praise God for the ability to smile and laugh at ourselves and our circumstances. Because He created us, He knows the emotional healing that comes from humor!

Support
I'm Giving You Your Smile Back

> *Let those who delight in my righteousness shout*
> *for joy and be glad and say evermore,*
> *"Great is the LORD, who delights in the welfare*
> *of His servant!"* Psalm 35:27

When Marilyn was diagnosed with ovarian cancer, time seemed to stand still. She and her husband just looked at each other in disbelief before they hugged and wept on the other's shoulder.

Then, a few short weeks after surgery to remove the tumor, Marilyn developed a blood clot in her leg. Walking back into the same hospital with another pain brought her fears and concerns to the surface. She was devastated by the addition of the complication, and depression began to set in. She wanted to be rid of all the pain and illness and negative feelings; she longed to have her old life back. Marilyn told her husband, "I just want my smile back!"

Hasn't everyone had those feelings at one time

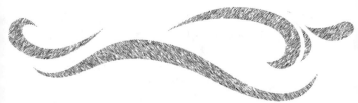

or another? God doesn't give us an escape pod so we can return to the life we once lived. And we can't know what's ahead, so we have to take each day as it comes. What comes isn't always of our choosing. But one thing is absolutely true—"God so loved the world, that He gave His only Son, that whoever believes in Him should not perish but have eternal life" (John 3:16). What joy we have with those words: God loves so much that He gave up His beloved Son just for us! It's the Gospel message in a nutshell.

When Christmas came that year, Marilyn's husband gave her a book he had made that celebrated each year of her life of 57 years. He titled it *57 Ways I Love You*. On the last page, he wrote, "I'm giving you your smile back." That gift sent Marilyn's heart singing with joy. In the same way, our hearts sing with joy when we remember the gift of eternal life we're given and the book that assures us of that life. Praise and all glory to Him!

Thanksgiving
Thank You, Lord

> *My lips will shout for joy, when I sing praises*
> *to You; my soul also, which You have redeemed.*
> Psalm 71:23

"Thank You, Lord, for this chair that lets me rest as I walk from the bedroom to the kitchen to get a glass of water. Oh, how good that cool water tastes! The fact that the chair is halfway between the two rooms provides relief when I lack strength. Just a few months ago, I would never have believed that I could be so weak that I could not walk that short way. But here I am. And I thank You, Lord, for allowing me just to be here," Linda prayed.

In Linda's life, it's the little things—like a drink of water and that convenient chair to sit on—that bring her joy. She loves the satiny feel of the chair cover. It's a luxury compared to the scratchy hospital linens. There's just something about satin that makes tender skin feel cool and comforted.

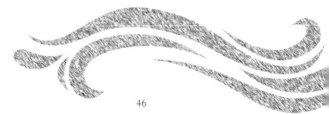

Taking a deep breath, Linda smells clean air. That's definitely a good thing! Nausea comes in waves when she smells certain things, even those she once dearly loved, such as the aroma of bread baking or the lemony scent of a clean house. How things change in a cancer survivor's life! She's been told that when she no longer has to endure chemotherapy, her nausea will disappear, and she will enjoy those wonderful aromas again.

Living in an apartment isn't the same as living in a house; other people infringe on your quiet time. Linda used to dislike hearing footsteps scampering above her. But that has changed for her too. Now, as she rests in her chair, she hears the children upstairs running to get ready for school. She imagines what they're doing—packing things in their backpacks, looking for a forgotten book, grabbing a quick recess snack. Then all is quiet again. She looks forward to their return from school so she can again imagine the children, fit and healthy, going about their lives in a lively way. It makes her smile.

Linda prayed, "I thank You, Lord, for the time to look around me and see—I mean really see. I am blessed to have a window in my bedroom that opens out on a grove of trees with bird feeders. I can watch the birds and laugh at their antics. I enjoy the tree branches swaying in the breeze. They bring a calm into my life and lull me into a restful nap. Thank You for my eyes, Lord. I enjoy my grandchildren's pictures. You know that my goal is to get stronger so that I can travel to see them.

"I praise You, Lord, for all the little things I notice now. My senses seem to be attuned to everything. I was so busy with 'life' before my cancer diagnosis that I missed a lot of what was going on around me. Now that I am forced to rest and slow down, I see, hear, touch, smell, and taste with a different perspective. I am so grateful! And more than that, I thank You, Father, for caring about me—caring so much that You gave Jesus to redeem me from sin and eternal death. How blessed I am because of Your love for me. Thank You, Jesus. Amen."

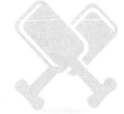

Witness
Coming Together

> *Then they cried to the LORD in their trouble,*
> *and He delivered them from their distress.*
> *He sent out His word and healed them,*
> *and delivered them from their destruction.*
> *Let them thank the LORD for His steadfast love,*
> *for His wondrous works to the children of man!*
> Psalm 107:19–21

It didn't take long to exhaust Barb's insurance coverage. Within weeks of her diagnosis of melanoma, she and her husband, Lee, had to make some hard choices about continuing her treatment. Barb felt guilty that her group policy covered so little of the experimental treatment that seemed to be working. Lee was desperate to do whatever it took to save Barb's life.

A temporary solution seemed to have a fundraiser. As soon as it was suggested, their friends took charge, planning a silent auction, dinner, and dance. A local catering company donated their time and provided the dinner at cost. A local band donated their time as well. An account was established at Barb's bank, and soon everyone was involved in getting the word out. And, God be praised, the fund-raiser was a success! More than three hundred people attended, and together they raised $37,000 to help with Barb's expenses.

Barb is the nurse at the town's middle school, so she knows hundreds of children and their parents. She also knows that her prognosis is not good. Barb's father had died of melanoma, and hers had metastasized to her liver before it was discovered. But she is determined that it not defeat her, so she willingly takes part in aggressive experimental treatment. "To me, this feels like a way I can try to beat my own cancer and help people who are diagnosed with it in the future," Barb says.

Because Barb works in a public school, she can't talk openly about her faith in Jesus as her Savior. But she knows that many of the students in her school go to church, and each time one of them tells her that they prayed for her in church or Sunday School, she says a heartfelt thank-you. "My witness to them is what means the most to me," Barb says. "It's those kids, the ones who know Jesus, who will understand that no matter what happens to me, God is faithful. They'll see my example of faith and it will, in turn, assure them of Christ's mercy and salvation."

Love
A Blessing in Disguise

And the King will answer them, "Truly, I say to you, as you did it to one of the least of these My brothers, you did it to Me." Matthew 25:40

Steve battled the despair he felt at being told he needed to have a laryngectomy. He didn't want to think about not being able to speak with his own voice box, or larynx. The oncologist first tried radiation and chemotherapy, hoping to preserve the larynx. But now it was clear that a laryngectomy was necessary to save Steve's earthly life.

51

Steve was a man of faith, and he trusted in Christ for his eternal life. But after surgery, Steve wanted nothing to do with therapy to learn to "talk." He had drain tubes and a hole in his neck. A big blue tube aimed at that hole provided humidified air. He couldn't see how he looked, but he could imagine it. And he was angry! Angry at the cancer that had come into his life. Angry that the radiation and chemo hadn't worked. Angry that he had a hole in his neck and no voice to speak. In his anger, Steve questioned why this had happened to him. But just as quickly he knew the answer: no one is devoid of problems.

First came a knock on the door, and then a head appeared. It was Thomas, a longtime friend and an elder at Steve's church. "Mind if I come in?" asked Thomas.

Steve motioned for him to come in. What else could he do? Thomas was his friend.

But *two* men walked in. Why is Thomas bringing someone else with him? This certainly is no time to meet someone new, Steve thought.

"Steve, I want to introduce you to my wife's cousin Hal. He and his family are on their way to Wyoming, and they stopped to visit us."

"Hi, Steve," said Hal.

Steve looked at Hal with surprise. There was something different about his voice.

"When Thomas told me he was going to visit you, I asked if I could come along," Hal said. "I had a laryngectomy a couple years ago, and I think I understand what you might be going through right now. Probably a lot of anger. Am I right?"

Steve nodded his head, affirming his emotional anger, but he couldn't take his eyes off of Hal.

Hal said, "Anger can slow down the process of healing and recovery. It's a normal emotion, but you don't want to dwell there too long. The important thing to do now is follow your doctor's plan for voice therapy. When you're able to communicate again, your emotional anger will begin to heal.

"Of course, the most important thing is talking with God," Hal continued. "Tell Him everything— your anger, your frustration, anything. He is your lifeline. Lean on Him as well as on your friends and family. They're all there for you, but you are the one who has to do the work. Keep at it! And know that God is right beside you, helping you every step of the way. Remember what Jesus said in John 16:33, 'In the world you will have tribulation. But take heart; I have overcome the world.' Steve, my faith grew stronger during my recovery, and I pray that you'll enjoy a stronger relationship with Him also. Okay?"

Again Steve nodded. His irritation turned to gratitude that Thomas had brought Hal to visit him. He began to be hopeful that he, too, could lead a functional life as Hal did.

Thomas prayed with him. And Hal gave Steve a strong handshake. "You'll do fine. I'm glad to have met you, Steve," said Hal.

A couple months later, Steve told Thomas what a wonderful blessing it had been that Hal visited him in the hospital. That conversation motivated him, and before Steve was released from the hospital, he had decided that he would visit other laryngectomy patients to offer the same kind of encouragement. As Hal said it would, Steve's faith in God's promises of forgiveness and salvation grew stronger. And prayer time is still an important part of each day. Hal was right—Steve's deeper faith in God may never have happened had it not been for his cancer. "And we know that for those who love God all things work together for good, for those who are called according to His purpose" (Romans 8:28).

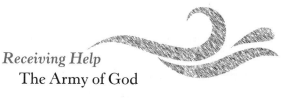

Receiving Help
The Army of God

> *From day to day men came to David*
> *to help him, until there was a great army,*
> *like an army of God.* 1 Chronicles 12:22

Joelle's cancer journey was terrifying at times, but also rewarding in many ways.

Rewarding? Oh, yes!

Her husband became her biggest cheerleader. Together, they met the challenges of life with cancer. He read all the literature and sought more information from every source he could find. Armed with good information, he became the head chef and dietitian during her chemotherapy and radiation treatments.

Joelle's boss became her anchor to sanity. After learning of her diagnosis, he arranged for her to work from home during her recovery from surgery. This was so important! She never felt that her job was in jeopardy. And during the chemo and radiation, she could still work at home when her energy level necessitated. She told her close friend, "My brain still works, even though my body is lacking its full power!"

There were some days that the chemo or radiation made her sick. But her co-workers were supportive and told her they would be glad to jump in and pick up the workload for her. They did just that! What a comfort to know life goes on when you're down for the count! It was a blessing that she didn't have to worry or feel guilty when she couldn't complete her work.

Joelle was amazed at the hundreds of cards, flowers, and gifts that were sent. She was so touched by the outpouring of affection and the offers of help. She said, "The prayers that were said for me were powerful. There were prayer chains and prayers in worship services. People I've never met prayed for me. I was humbled, but uplifted at the same time. I had the whole army of God surrounding me and battling this cancer right beside me."

Yes, cancer can be rewarding when you have the whole army of God surrounding you, cheering you on, helping you in your battle, lifting you up when you fall down. All praise and glory to God, who knows the needs of each one of us and provides us with the help and comfort we need!

Holidays
Holiday Surprises

> *The saying is trustworthy and deserving of full acceptance, that Christ Jesus came into the world to save sinners, of whom I am the foremost.* 1 Timothy 1:15

"What's wrong, Julie?" asked her mother, Michelle.

"Sorry, Mom. I'm just sad."

"Tell me why," Michelle said as she sat down on the bed beside her daughter.

Julie took a deep breath and said, "Tomorrow is December 1, and I won't be able to do anything fun to prepare for Christmas."

"I know, Sweetie, but when you finish the chemo and get stronger, we'll look forward to those Advent preparations and Christmas shopping trips, won't we?"

Michelle hugged her and then went downstairs to finish lunch, all the while wondering what she could do to help her thirteen-year-old daughter, who was undergoing treatments for leukemia.

Julie hadn't fussed over her treatments; she knew how important they were. But Michelle knew that Julie was lonely, and she wanted to help ease her sadness. Suddenly, a thought began to take shape.

The next day was Saturday, and the rest of the family surprised Julie at breakfast. They presented her with a large gift box wrapped in Christmas paper and tied with red and green ribbons. Michelle; Julie's dad, Ken; and her brother and sister, Paul and Anna, watched Julie open the box. Inside were twenty-four smaller boxes. Each small box was also wrapped in pretty Christmas paper, and the boxes were numbered from 1 to 24.

"Wow!" exclaimed Julie. "What are all these?"

Ken said, "We know that this year you can't do some of the fun things you like to do during Advent and Christmas, so we created some fun for you."

Michelle continued, "At breakfast each morning in December, you can open one gift. In it might be something we'll do together that day, or it might be just a little something fun for you to do on your own."

"Yeah," added Anna, "we all came up with fun ideas for your box."

Paul said, "Today you get to open box number 1."

"This is so much fun!" cried Julie as she began to unwrap the box. Inside were four decorated sheets of paper with the names Dad, Mom, Paul, and Anna on them. Each person had selected an activity that would occupy Julie's time for one hour. Dad wanted to play board games with her. Mom wanted Julie to help with ideas for Christmas gifts for family and friends; they would check online for costs and availability. Paul challenged her to a game of chess. And Anna wanted to begin their "special project" for Mom and Dad—the ready-to-paint crèche figures they had already purchased.

"Thank you for your special gifts. It's great to be in this family. Thanks for helping me enjoy the

Advent season as part of the family. I'd like my life to be what it was before leukemia—and I hope that it will be again someday—but I wouldn't want to go through this with anyone else but you."

That night, as Julie got ready for bed, she tested the paint on the figurines she and Anna had painted earlier. All were dry. Lovingly, she touched baby Jesus last. "How special You are, Jesus! You bring such peace to my life, knowing You are with me through all my tests and pain. I love thinking about how You came to earth with such purpose! Mom says You are the world's first Christmas present! To think that You came to die for me and everyone so we could be forgiven and go to heaven. That's awesome! Thank You, Jesus! Thank You for my family!"

Julie yawned and closed her eyes. Visions of what the second box would bring the next morning danced in her head, but her hand still clutched baby Jesus near to her heart as she drifted off to sleep.

Hope
Sharing Hope

> *I can do all things through Him*
> *who strengthens me.* Philippians 4:13

Five years after Kevin was diagnosed with lung cancer, he rejoiced that he was a five-year survivor. Today, he's still rejoicing—and he celebrates forty-three years of being cancer-free.

Kevin's town has an annual "race" for cancer survivors. It doesn't matter what kind of cancer the people had. They just walk or run for the sheer joy of being with others who have been on their own cancer journey. He is always impressed by how many people participate, marveling at the number of volunteers and sponsors who make the event so special for everyone. He looks forward to it every year.

Kevin has become something of a celebrity at this event. Each year, he attaches a ribbon to his ball cap for another year that he has been blessed to be cancer-free. When he talks with others about surviving lung cancer, their eyes widen in awe when they learn how many years it's been. Year after year at this event, Kevin spreads hope as he shows how healthy and energetic cancer survivors can be.

But Kevin is quick to explain that his real hope—and ours—comes from the One who heals us of all pain and sorrow. Paul's Letter to the Romans reminds us that we are alive to God in Christ (6:11), that we have eternal life as a free gift in Christ (6:23). For in Christ Jesus, we "consider that the sufferings of this present time are not worth comparing with the glory that is to be revealed to us" (Romans 8:18).

Throughout life, the believer runs the race with faith in Christ. He is our hope!

Strength
The War in My Mind

*For the sake of Christ, then, I am content with
weaknesses, insults, hardships, persecutions, and
calamities. For when I am weak, then I am strong.*
2 Corinthians 12:10

Carly's life with melanoma hasn't been fun.
"Cancer is the worst thing that ever happened to
me," she says. "But cancer is also the best thing that
ever happened to me."

How can one person have such opposing
thoughts?

Carly says, "Cancer is the
pits! The treatments made me
sick and weak. My tastes and
smells changed, and my hair
fell out. Even my eyebrows and
eyelashes fell out. Now, how can
a young woman get past that!
Nevertheless there's one good
thing about losing my hair . . .
my hair dryer and curling iron
got a much-needed rest.

Knowing the pain and suffering that Jesus went through, I am certain that He understands my pain.

"Cancer has been a blessing in my life too! I think about all the amazing people I've met and the good changes that have affected my life. If there's one thing I've learned, it's to trust those who are more knowledgeable than I am. The doctors and nurses are wonderful—so compassionate and supportive!"

Carly's faith in Christ Jesus brought her through the challenges. She doesn't hesitate to tell others how much stronger she feels when she gets to the other side of a bad day. "I have learned that when I am weakest, then my faith is strongest. I may have a terrible day, but my daily Bible readings and prayer lift me up and fill me with contentment. Knowing the pain and suffering that Jesus went through, I am certain that He understands my pain. And because I have faith, I know Jesus is by my side through all the treatments and subsequent effects of those treatments."

Cancer has given Carly new opportunities to serve her Lord. As she shares her story with other people at the cancer center, she is able to lift them up with hope and encouragement. She is an advocate for education and healthy living; Carly speaks out on using sunscreen and avoiding tanning beds.

She continues, "I'm not happy that I am back with treatments for the second time; however, the support and encouragement from my friends and medical team is wonderful. They make me smile, and I know that a positive attitude is important for my recovery and my outlook on life. But more than that, trusting in God's plan of salvation for me sustains me through the tough times."

Praise Him!

I know that a positive
attitude is important
for my recovery
and my outlook on life.
Praise Him!

Support
Just What I Needed!

*Our help is in the name of the Lord,
who made heaven and earth. Psalm 124:8*

Nina had recently gone through a painful divorce. She worked full-time and had an eleven-year-old son. Then, when she was only forty-six, she received the news that she had cancer: ductal carcinoma in situ (DCIS), a common, noninvasive type of breast cancer.

Cancer was no stranger—her mother had died of pancreatic cancer—and Nina was determined to fight the disease. The plan was for a lumpectomy, radiation, and then an extended time of medication. Although she had to factor in a five-days-a-week treatment schedule, Nina thought she could do it all. At first. She quickly learned that she couldn't handle the stress on her own; she needed help with her emotions.

Nina sought out a therapist with whom she felt comfortable enough to be honest and open. Having this outlet gave her renewed emotional strength and the ability to look to the future with a positive attitude.

Her therapist encouraged her to join a group for cancer support activities and services. Through that group, Nina learned about the wide array of free services available to her. For example, she visited a resource library that provided valuable information about the aspects of living with cancer. She took part in nutrition workshops and free exercise classes, and she joined a support group. Being able to talk about problems and frustrations with people who understood the emotions she was feeling was uplifting and meaningful. Eventually, Nina took on the role of overseeing the cancer support group in her own area as a way of "paying it forward."

Nina is recovering from cancer. She is excited about her future and helping others cope. She continues to rely on her Lord and Savior Jesus Christ as her source of hope and joy. Through her experience, she has become a blessing to everyone she meets because she helps them rely on Him too.

Support

Words Have Different Meanings to Different People

> *My heart throbs; my strength fails me,*
>   *and the light of my eyes—*
>   *it also has gone from me.*
> *My friends and companions stand aloof*
>   *from my plague, and my nearest kin*
>   *stand far off. . . .*
> *Do not forsake me, O LORD!*
>   *O my God, be not far from me!*
> *Make haste to help me,*
>   *O Lord, my salvation!*
>   Psalm 38:10–11, 21–22

Willa ran into her friend Kathy at the grocery store. Kathy was recovering from lung cancer; Willa was recovering from breast cancer. The two spent several minutes sharing stories about people who say the most outrageous things. For instance, because Kathy had a lung removed, she becomes winded easily; she has a handicapped placard in

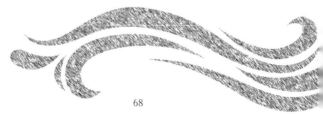

her car so she can park closer to her destinations. Kathy said, "Someone actually told me I was fortunate to be able to park in a handicapped spot. I would much rather be healthy and able to walk from the farthest corner of the parking lot!"

Willa told about the times people have said, "You look so good! Doesn't she look good?" She continued, "Why are people so surprised that I look okay because I have cancer? They've even said it when I felt terribly sick! I asked my husband why some people were saying this to me. He said he didn't know, but with the changes we've made in our diet, he thinks I really do look better now. I'll take that as a compliment!" Both of them laughed.

Kathy and Willa concluded that perhaps they're sensitive to the words of well-meaning people because cancer is an emotional topic. Willa confessed, "I have to admit that before I knew what it was like to have cancer, I probably said some awkward things to others too. You know the saying 'Don't judge someone until you've walked a mile in his shoes.'"

As they said their good-byes, Kathy said, "I am glad we ran into each other, Willa. It's so good to talk to someone who understands. I talk to God a lot and ask Him to give me 'tough skin' and a forgiving heart so the unthinking remarks of others don't hurt so much. I'm getting better about it. And I believe that through this, God is using me as an instrument of His love."

"Oh, Kathy," Willa said, "you are definitely that. I've said many prayers about the same thing. I fight the urge to shout at them, to tell them that I just want to hear that they love me or that they're praying for me! Prayer is what I need; that's what we all need. I'm so glad I bumped into you, Kathy. Take care and God's blessings to you!"

Prayer
Prayer Connection

> *Do not be anxious about anything,*
> *but in everything by prayer and supplication*
> *with thanksgiving let your requests*
> *be made known to God.* Philippians 4:6

Lindsay stood by the big bay window in the breakfast nook and looked out at the falling snow. Her good friend Nina was in the kitchen, fixing coffee. Lindsay asked, "Nina, do you remember when we were young and there were times when we wanted something so much that we would hold each other's hands and pray as hard as we could?"

Nina, carrying two steaming cups of coffee, came and stood by Lindsay. "Yes, I remember," she said, handing her friend a mug and lifting it in salute. "Those were the days, weren't they? So carefree. Back then, we never would have believed that we'd be standing here today toasting our one-year anniversary of being cancer-free."

Lindsay took a sip and then said, "As I was going through the chemo and radiation, I prayed a lot. It was just me and the IV bag or me and the x-ray machine. I would think about how fervently we prayed together when we were younger, and it helped to quiet my fears. I am so glad to have you as part of that foundation."

"I know just what you're talking about," Nina said. "I, too, treasure the memories of our praying together. That really was a special time. We still have that connection, don't we? It's a joy to me that we still pray with and for each other."

"It is," Lindsay agreed. "You're my best friend and prayer partner. Let's pray together now."

Clasping the handle of a coffee cup with one hand and her best friend's hand with the other, each woman bowed her head and went to God in prayer, as she had so many times throughout their years of friendship.

Lindsay: "Oh, heavenly Father, we praise and thank You for Your presence in our lives. What would we do without Your Word of promise and comfort? You are a constant comfort to us in everything we face every day. Keep us ever in your care, Lord. And continue to be with our families. Send Your Spirit to help them face their fears. Strengthen their faith and help them to put their trust in You."

Nina: "Yes, Father, take care of our loved ones. They are so special to us and, oh, how we need them. Your love gives us strength and peace to sustain us through all of our treatment and recovery. If it be Your will, Lord, free us of this disease. In Your precious Son's name we ask it. Amen.

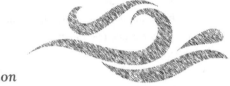

Depression
Support from Those Who Know

> In my distress I called upon the Lord;
> to my God I cried for help.
> From His temple He heard my voice,
> and my cry to Him reached His ears.
> Psalm 18:6

It's very difficult to hear a life-threatening diagnosis. Most cancer patients say that's the worst part of the journey. Take Tyler. His everyday life was disrupted, and he needed to learn to walk to the beat of a new drummer. He felt angry because his life had been turned upside down with the news that he had bone cancer, and somehow he had to learn how to make the abnormal into his new normal. Tyler knew that sometimes just having cancer can lead to depression, but he felt he was strong enough emotionally to avoid that side effect.

But bone cancer is painful, and Tyler was physically uncomfortable. Pain can worsen symptoms of depression, leading to feelings of hopelessness and lack of self-worth.

Tyler's doctor recognized his malaise and suggested that he participate in the hospital Guided Imagery program. "They'll teach you how to relax and use progressive muscle relaxation in an effort to relax the mind, reduce pain, and decrease anxiety."

Tyler tried the meetings and loved them. He said, "My family is great and loves me so much; however, I know that every person in that group knows and understands the emotional part of cancer. That means so much to me. It's like we're all in it together and support one another.

"I attend church every week, go to Sunday School, and meet with my weekly Bible study group. I thought I was doing as well as could be expected. I guess I needed a little more. My doctor knew that extra support was just what I needed in addition to my loving Savior, who provides for my every need."

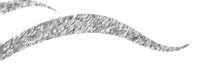

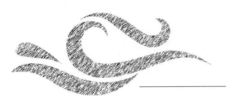

_____

_____

_____

_____

_____

_____

_____

_____

_____

_____

_____

_____

_____

_____

_____

_____

_____

_____

_____

Prayers

Do not be anxious
about anything,

but in everything by prayer
and supplication

with thanksgiving
let your requests
be made known to God.

Philippians 4:6

God invites us and expects us to pray in Jesus' name. We are free to go to Him at all times and in all places because Jesus reconciled us to God and intercedes on our behalf. Prayer is a gift from God to us as His children. And our heavenly Father promises to listen and to answer.

Prayer helps us to keep God's will in front of us. He knows what is best for us. That is why we pray to ask him to bring us in line with His Word and His will for us.

When Jesus' disciples asked about the proper way to pray, He gave them the model for prayer, which we call the Lord's Prayer. All forms of prayer—confession, adoration, thanksgiving, intercession—are based on this perfect model.

God calls us to the joyous responsibility and privilege of regular, confident conversation with Him. Perhaps you already have the habit of daily prayer. If not, this very day is the perfect time to begin. In either case, may the prayers in this book be a blessing to you and to those for whom you pray.

A model for daily prayer

Invocation: In the name of the Father and of the Son and of the Holy Spirit. Amen.

Hymn: Beginning on page 157 is a selection of hymns chosen to bless you during your devotion time.

Scripture reading: Throughout all of Scripture, God teaches about life on earth, death, and life everlasting. A few passages, beginning on page 125, have been chosen for you.

Devotional reading: Each devotion deals with a topic unique to those who are dealing with cancer. Devotions are featured on pages 11 to 74.

Prayer: Use the brief prayers in this section to conclude your time of meditation and as you need them throughout your day.

General Prayers

The Lord's Prayer

Our Father who art in heaven,
hallowed be Thy name,
Thy kingdom come,
Thy will be done on earth as it is in heaven;
give us this day our daily bread;
and forgive us our trespasses as we forgive
those who trespass against us;
and lead us not into temptation,
but deliver us from evil,
For Thine is the kingdom and the power
and the glory forever and ever. Amen.

Morning Prayer

I thank You, my heavenly Father, through Jesus Christ, Your dear Son, that You have kept me this night from all harm and danger; and I pray that You would keep me this day also from sin and every evil, that all my doings and life may please You. For into Your hands I commend myself, my body and soul, and all things. Let Your holy angel be with me, that the evil foe may have no power over me. Amen. (LUTHER'S MORNING PRAYER)

Prayer at Midday

Lord God, heavenly Father, You watched over the Israelites in a cloud by day and a pillar of fire by night. Continue to watch over me, my family, friends, and caregivers as this day continues. Even though cancer has invaded my body, which You have created, nothing can ever remove Your love from me through Your Son, Jesus. There is nowhere I can go from Your presence. You are all-seeing, all-knowing, all-powerful. How great is Your faithfulness. I rest confidently in Your love. Amen.

(PORTALS OF PRAYER)

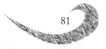

Evening Prayer

I thank You, my heavenly Father, through Jesus Christ, Your dear Son, that You have graciously kept me this day; and I pray that You would forgive me all my sins where I have done wrong, and graciously keep me this night. For into Your hands I commend myself, my body and soul, and all things. Let Your holy angel be with me, that the evil foe may have no power over me. Amen. (LUTHER'S EVENING PRAYER)

Prayer at Midnight

Heavenly Father, as another day quietly begins in the midst of darkness, I offer to You my praise and adoration. While many people sleep at this hour, I rejoice that You neither slumber nor sleep and that You are always ready to hear my prayers for healing. For the sake of Your Son, Jesus Christ, the light of the world, scatter the darkness that exists in my life. Forgive my sins, remove all my doubts, comfort me in my sorrows, and take away all my fears and anxieties. Grant Your blessings on this new day, that all I think, say, and do may please You. In Jesus' name I pray. Amen. (PORTALS OF PRAYER)

Mealtime Prayers

Lord God, heavenly Father,
bless us and these Your gifts,
which we receive from
Your bountiful goodness,
through Jesus Christ,
our Lord. Amen.

Heavenly Father, we thank You for the gift of food You have provided and for all those whose labor brings Your blessings to our table. We pray that at this meal we may be strengthened for Your service and together may await with joy the feast You have prepared for all the faithful in Your eternal kingdom; through Jesus Christ, our Lord. Amen. (*LSB*, p. 315)

Returning Thanks

Give thanks to the Lord, for He is good. His love endures forever. He gives food to every creature. He provides food for the cattle and for the young ravens when they call. His pleasure is not in the strength of the horse, nor His delight in the legs of a man; the Lord delights in those who fear Him, who put their hope in His unfailing love. Amen. (PSALM 136:1, 25; 147:9–11 NIV)

We thank You, Lord God, heavenly Father, for all Your benefits, through Jesus Christ, our Lord, who lives and reigns with You and the Holy Spirit forever and ever. Amen. (Adapted from Luther's Small Catechism)

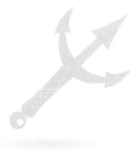

Sunday

Heavenly Father, on this first day of a new week, You awaken me to a new celebration of Your Son's glorious resurrection victory. Grant me again the assurance and promise of my own resurrection as Your baptized and forgiven child. Fill my heart with gladness in Your precious promises, and give me true zeal for Your holy house on this day of rest. Prepare me in humility and faith to hear Your Holy Word and to receive Your precious Sacrament. Console me with Your word of Absolution. Strengthen my faith and my body to fight cancer. If it is Your will, restore me to full health. My trust is in You. In Jesus' name. Amen. (*PORTALS OF PRAYER*)

Monday

Gracious God and heavenly Father, I thank You for Your loving care and presence in my life. Your love and faithfulness will carry me through each day because Your mercy in Christ will never end. Restore my energy to fulfill all that You have planned for me today. Forgive me when I get discouraged and want to give up. Great Physician, bring healing to my body. Give me clarity in vision to see the blessings You continually give me and then boldly speak about these blessings with others. I rest secure in my relationship with Jesus Christ, who died for my sins, endured the cross, and rose again for me. Amen.

Tuesday

Heavenly Father, Your mercies are new to me every day. Open my eyes to recognize the many blessings You have given me. Enable me to see the people You place before me today who care for me and who help me find comfort from the side effects of treatments. Fill me with gratitude for all You do for me. Make me aware that by responding in love to others, in spite of my afflictions, I am serving You. In Christ Jesus I pray. Amen. (PORTALS OF PRAYER)

Wednesday

Almighty God, thank You for sanctifying me this day for Jesus' sake because He has saved me by His life, death, and resurrection. You provide for all my needs of body and soul. Forgive me when I worry about the test results and spend sleepless nights concerned about my future. Rescue me from the fiery attacks of Satan, who seeks to discourage me and weaken my faith. Today I lay my burdens at the foot of the cross. Secure in me the knowledge of Your love and Christ's sacrifice for me. By Your mercy, lead me to rejoice all the more in the salvation You freely give me for Jesus' sake. Amen.

Thursday

Lord God Almighty, I begin this day with many uncertainties. Will I be able to endure the trials of this disease today? You know the plans You have for me, plans to prosper me and not to harm me, plans to give me hope and a future. It is great comfort to my soul that You always want the best for me. Nothing is impossible for You. I look at situations from human eyes with limitations. You have no boundaries. How grateful I am that I can trust You with my life. In mercy, bring healing to my brokenness according to Your holy and gracious will. In Jesus' name. Amen.

Friday

Dear Lord, by Your grace I have another day to glorify You. At home, doctor offices, support groups, and with my family and friends, use me to reflect Your love. May others see in me the hope I have in trusting You through the changes and challenges that come with cancer. Let Your Spirit fill me with patience and understanding as I deal with unexpected situations. From Your presence, engulf me with the peace that transcends all understanding. You live and reign with the Father and the Holy Spirit, one God, now and forever. Amen. (PORTALS OF PRAYER)

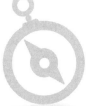

Saturday

Heavenly Father, I come into Your presence this day with heartfelt gratitude for the undeserved blessings of Your goodness. I confess that I have offended You in word and deed. With a contrite heart, I ask You to forgive my sins for the sake of Jesus, who paid for them with His divine and precious blood. Send Your holy angels to watch over me and my loved ones. Grant me quiet rest under the shadow of Your wing. Keep my loved ones under Your protection and in steadfast faith in Christ. Grant those who suffer from cancer and other illnesses rest from pain and sorrow. Give us all peace and rest through Your dear Son, Jesus, in whose name we pray. Amen. (PORTALS OF PRAYER)

For Blessings on the Word

Lord God, bless Your Word where it is proclaimed. Make it a Word of power and peace to convert those not yet Your own and to confirm those who have come to saving faith. May Your Word pass from the ear to the heart and from the heart to the lips. May the words of my heart achieve that purpose for which You sent them; through Jesus Christ, my Lord. Amen. (*PORTALS OF PRAYER*)

For Divine Guidance

Holy Lord, You have revealed the way to salvation and life through the illuminating Word of Scripture. Help me to understand your desires for my life as I read Your Holy Word. Make it a light to guide me, knowing Your faithfulness will sustain me through cancer and all the challenges. Grant that the truths revealed therein might sharpen my resolve to follow Your perfect will. Open the way for me to follow You, my Great Shepherd. Amen. (*PORTALS OF PRAYER*)

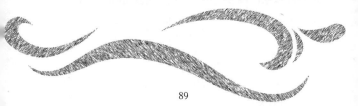

For Faithful Reception of the Lord's Supper

What a blessing You give me when I receive the Lord's Supper! Through this Sacrament, I receive with the bread and wine the body and blood of my Savior Jesus Christ! My sins are forgiven, and my faith in Christ as my Lord and Savior is daily strengthened. Help me to be faithful in receiving Your Sacrament. In Your name, Jesus, I ask it. Amen. (*PORTALS OF PRAYER*)

For Faithfulness under the Cross

Father, as You helped Your Son as He walked the way of sorrows carrying His cross, comfort and strengthen me as I bear my cross. Keep me from losing faith in this time of testing, and increase my trust in you even more. Help me to believe that You are at work through this trial, and cause me to remember "that the sufferings of this present time are not worth comparing with the glory that is to be revealed" (Romans 8:18). I pray in Jesus' name. Amen. (*PORTALS OF PRAYER*)

For the Peace of Christ

Prince of Peace, continue to give me the certain assurance that only in You can I experience in my daily life a peace "which surpasses all understanding" (Philippians 4:7). Give me this peace, which results from Your suffering, death, and resurrection for me. By Your undeserved love, my sins are forgiven. You are my Lord, and I am Your child. Help me to look to You alone for strength and peace during my cancer journey. Amen. (*PORTALS OF PRAYER*)

Topical Prayers

Acceptance

Heavenly Father, I was not prepared to hear the tests results. I felt numb, weak, and devastated. Sustain me through Your Word, where I find comfort for my heart and Your faithfulness in all circumstances! Whatever is in store for me, give me courage and strength to accept this trial, an understanding mind, a surrendered will, and everlasting hope. I claim Your promises: You will *never* forsake me, with You all things are possible, You bring good from the painful and unexpected. Your ultimate sacrifice for me on the cross is my salvation and peace. In the name of Jesus, my Savior. Amen.

Anxiety

Merciful Father, thank You for the privilege of coming to You just as I am and the assurance that You will always listen as I pour out my honest thoughts and feelings. I'm angry that my life has changed so drastically. I'm scared about the unknown. My thoughts go from suffering and side effects to financial pressure and my own mortality. Have mercy on me; forgive me for my lack of trust in You. Calm my anxious heart, dear Lord. Help me to learn to live one day at a time. You are my Rock and my Refuge. In Jesus' name. Amen.

Appearance

Dear Father, I question my worth when I look in the mirror. My hair swept away in the garbage leaves me naked, vulnerable, and scared. Your Word assures me that real beauty comes from Your presence within me, and yet I battle discouragement. Help me to focus not on what cancer is doing to my physical body, but on how You are remaking and molding the inside of me. You are the foundation of my worth. Your love for me is irrevocable! I rejoice knowing that someday when I am in heaven, I will have the perfect body and be pain-free. What a glorious day that will be! In the name of Jesus. Amen.

Assurance

All-knowing Father, You oversee every detail of my life. Although I do not know what each day will bring, You do. I rest in the confidence that You will never forsake me and that I am not to be afraid. Your promises never fail! This security engulfs me with strength and courage. Nothing, neither death nor life, nor anything in all creation, will be able to separate me from the love of God in Christ Jesus. You are my stability in so much change that is happening in my life. I praise You for the gift of eternal life! In the name of Jesus, my Savior. Amen.

Attitude

Eternal Father, I'm consumed with the many negatives about suffering from cancer, such as side effects of medications that leave me exhausted and unable to think clearly. Grant me clear vision to see the many positive things from cancer. Cancer will never take Your love away from me! Cancer cannot shatter my hope in You! Cancer cannot keep You from forgiving my sins and giving me eternal life! I'm assured, from Your Word, that my inner attitudes do not have to reflect outward circumstances. Help me to have a positive perspective and a Christ-centered attitude. Thank You, Lord! Amen.

Baptismal Grace

Lord Jesus Christ, You came in humility and weakness to defeat the powers of sin, death, and the devil. Clothe our weaknesses with Your righteousness by Your baptismal grace, that we might withstand the power of every adversary; for You live and reign with the Father and the Holy Spirit, one God, now and forever. Amen. (*VISITATION*, p. 57)

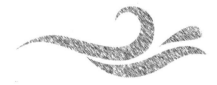

Birthday

Lord, this is the day You have made, and I rejoice and am glad in it. As I celebrate another year of life, I thank You for knitting me together in my mother's womb, for giving me countless blessings, and for providing for all my needs of body and soul. I especially praise you for the new life You gave me in Baptism, for the gift of the Gospel, and for the bounty of Your grace. Bless all my tomorrows with Your favor. In Jesus' name I pray. Amen. (*PORTALS OF PRAYER*)

By a Hospice Worker

Almighty God, heavenly Father, as You have taken my life and made it holy in the death of Your Son, Jesus Christ, so, too, take the labor of my hands into Your own holy hands to accomplish Your will. Strengthen me in my work so discouragement, anger, and sadness do not overtake me, but that all I do may be pleasing in Your sight; through Jesus Christ, Your Son, our Lord. Amen. (*BLESSINGS*, p. 30)

Chemo Treatments

Ever-caring Savior, I confess that I'm not very brave these days. The rude intruders of nausea and weakness from diarrhea and mouth sores leave me depressed. Keep me mindful that chemo will kill the cancerous cells. Grant me victory over weakness and discouragement. Help me to concentrate on the treatments I've finished, not how many I have yet to go. Restore my spirit by Your presence. I will never be alone. You suffered and endured the cross for the joy set before me. Help me to endure the side effects for the hopeful healing and with assurance that eternal life is mine. In Jesus' name. Amen.

Decisions

Lord God, almighty Counselor, because You know everything, You know the decisions before me and the way I should go. I want only Your will, Lord. I no longer have the choice of waiting, so I will choose one of the options. If this decision is not right in Your sight, I ask Your Holy Spirit to put a heaviness in my heart. If this is the right direction for me to take, please confirm it with Your peace. I am willing to take whatever detours You decide to put in my path, as long as I reach the destination You have for me. I am in Your hands. In Christ's precious name I pray. Amen. (*BLESSINGS*, p. 39)

Distressed

Lord God eternal, by Your grace we live, and by Your mercy we are redeemed. Look on me in my distress and pain, and take from me the challenges of today. In Your love, let me find inner peace; in Your Word, hope for healing; in Your promises, consolation. Let Your presence protect me and Your mercies remove all anxiety and cares. Graciously forgive me all my sins. Keep me in Your loving care because of Him who died that I might live. In Christ Jesus, my Savior. Amen. (*VISITATION*, p. 4)

Doctors and Professional Health-Care Workers

Ever-caring Savior and Great Physician, I am grateful for the doctors, nurses, and other health-care workers who care for me. Give them clarity in thought, discernment, and wisdom to make the best choices for my treatment and healing. Bless them with patience and perseverance when they are overwhelmed from the stress of dealing daily with illness. I praise You, that in the midst of my cancer journey I can securely rest in Your grace. If it is according to Your good will and pleasure, restore me to health of body and mind. Through Jesus Christ, my Lord. Amen.

It was no accident that I have the compassionate doctors and nurses who care for me.

Encouraging Words

Lord Jesus, You know exactly when I need to hear encouraging words! I rejoiced when I heard "The tests show there are no new cells." "I'll see you in six months." I'm comforted through cards and phone calls. Thank You for using others to boost my spirit and for those who raise persistent prayers on my behalf. Forgive me when I have the opportunity to encourage others and I fail. Fill me with Your Spirit to share my faith and talk about the peace that comes through knowing "God so loved the world, that He gave His only Son, that whoever believes in Him should not perish but have eternal life" (John 3:16). Amen.

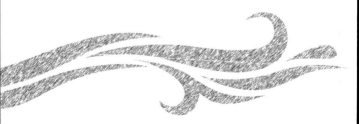

Governing Lord, I've come to another fork in the road with another aggressive chemotherapy. Only You know if it will be successful. Help me to rejoice in Your faithfulness to past generations and to me, and send Your Holy Spirit to guide me to trust You right now. You were with Joseph in the pit, Daniel in the lions' den, Sarah when she doubted, and Moses as he stepped out in faith to cross the Red Sea. Whenever I feel overwhelmed from little things like no taste to my food to big things like intense pain, bring my thoughts back to Your Word, Your faithfulness in every circumstance, and Your Son's precious life given for mine. Thank You for the encouragement and strength I find as I read, "I lift up my eyes to the hills. From where does my help come? My help comes from the LORD, who made heaven and earth. He will not let your foot be moved; He who keeps you will not slumber. . . . The LORD is your keeper; the LORD is your shade on your right hand. . . . The LORD will keep your going out and your coming in from this time forth and forevermore" (Psalm 121:1–3, 5, 8). To You be all glory, honor, and praise. Amen.

Family

God of love, I come to you with concerns for my family. A positive diagnosis of cancer is a shock to the whole family system. They are scared and hurt because I hurt. Shelter them from any repercussions of my disease, Lord. We look to You to lead us safely through the unknown days ahead. Grant us patience. Strengthen us by Your Holy Word. Nourish us with Christ's body and blood, and bring us safely to our eternal home. In the name of the Father, Son, and Holy Spirit. Amen.

Fear

Almighty Provider, there are many uncertainties in my life, and I am afraid. What will the long-term effect from radiation be? Will the cancer spread? Will I see my grandchildren grow up? Sovereign Lord, pour down on me the abundance of Your mercy. Forgive me those things of which my conscience is afraid, and give me those good things of which I am not worthy. Teach me to be still and know that You are God. You cover me with Your feathers; under Your wings I find refuge. I desire to make You my dwelling place. In Your refuge no harm will befall me. Thank You, Lord. Amen.

Feeling Helpless

Holy Jesus, wonderful Savior, eternal Lord, amid the anxieties of life and the sufferings of today, I seek refuge in You. You alone can give me the strength and endurance necessary to survive the day. In Your grace, protect me from all danger. Wash me thoroughly from my sin. Put a wall of love and trust around me to protect my heart from doubt and worry. Enfold me in Your forgiving arms because of Christ Jesus, my Savior. Amen. (*Visitation*, p. 22)

Finances

Faithful Father, I need Your holy guidance to help me through this maze. Prescriptions and medical treatments are rising, and my limited income is not enough anymore. All along Your sustaining hand has been with me, and Your grace is always sufficient. Help me to continue to find new paths of financial help. Keep me mindful that the ravens have no storehouse, and yet You feed them. There is security in knowing that I am more valuable to You than the birds. That empowers me with hope! I acknowledge that Your grace will always be sufficient! My total dependence is on You. In Jesus' name I pray. Amen.

Finances

Heavenly Counselor, You know I cannot work because of my cancer, and my spouse is out of work too. We haven't finished paying off the bills from before. How will we survive financially? How will we manage? Father, forgive my doubt. Keep me mindful of Your faithfulness to us in the past and of how You always provide for us in ways we least expect. Through Your grace, I will continue to believe in You and the precious promises of Your Word. Help me always to remember that the just will live by their faith in You. Thank You for blessing us with abundance and prosperity at Your timing, not ours. In Jesus' name. Amen.

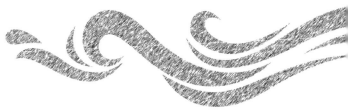

Friends

My Savior, my Friend, thank You for the blessing of committed friends and family. They listen while I laugh, cry, and express intense emotions. They offer silent companionship when I have no energy. They are a tangible expression of Your presence and love. This is much more than I deserve. You have blessed and strengthened me with new friends when I take treatments. Use me to be their friend too. It was no accident that I have compassionate doctors and nurses who care for me. You, my Friend, arrange even the most insignificant details in my day. To You be all glory, honor, and praise. Amen.

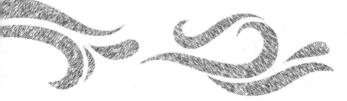

God's Promises

Precious Father, I've learned that all cancers have in common varying emotional reactions—mood swings. I'm not the only one aware of the changes in my emotions. My family, friends, and co-workers are aware as well. Even the people at the grocery store know when I'm having a bad day.

I find peace in Your Word, Lord, and when I read what You say to me in the pages of my Bible, I have more control over my mood swings. Help me to make it a priority to read Your Word daily, because this is where inner peace grows and calms my anxious heart. Your Word is my personal GPS: God's Promises for the Storm:

"But He said to me, 'My grace is sufficient for you, for My power is made perfect in weakness.' Therefore I will boast all the more gladly of my weaknesses, so that the power of Christ may rest upon me" (2 Corinthians 12:9). "And the peace of God, which surpasses all understanding, will guard your hearts and your minds in Christ Jesus" (Philippians 4:7). "Peace I leave with you; My peace I give you. Not as the world gives do I give to you.

Let not your hearts be troubled, neither let them be afraid" (John 14:27).

I rest in Your holy arms, Lord, because You love me and Your promises are forever. In Jesus' name. Amen.

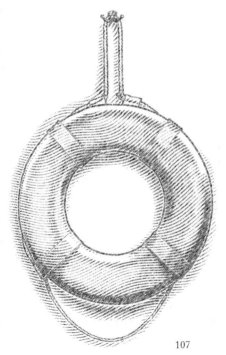

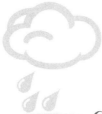

Good Days—Bad Days

Precious Jesus, my journey through cancer is filled with good days and really tough ones. When the doctors finally get the right combination of drugs and I'm not sick anymore, I rejoice. But when the blood count doesn't come back right and I can't take the treatment, I am brokenhearted. Graciously remind me that You promise to work all things, my good days and tough times, for good for those who love You. Clothe my weakness with Your baptismal grace. My hope is in You, who died for my sins and rose again so that I might have eternal life. Amen.

Guidance

My heavenly Father and my best Friend, I am in remission. Thank You, Lord! The doctors won't remove the port yet, but I'm hoping that will happen soon because it is uncomfortable—especially when people hug me. I so welcome their affection, but how do I let them know hugging is uncomfortable for me at this time? You have promised to be my Guide until I die, and that includes guiding me through big things like living with cancer as well as little things like hugs. You are my personal Guidance Counselor. Help me to listen when You speak and then obediently follow where Your Word leads me. I praise You, Holy Father! Amen.

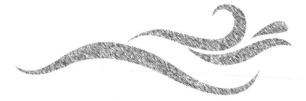

Almighty Counselor, You promise guidance and wisdom to all who ask for it. I'm overwhelmed with the decisions I need to make: How radical should my treatments be? What are the implications for the kind of surgery I choose? Should I have genetic testing? This is such new territory. I'm humbled and humiliated to feel so inadequate. I know I cannot do this alone. Father, I praise You for inviting me to lay all my burdens at Your feet. Help me to be still and sensitive to Your nudges. Let me rest in the comfort of Your divine guidance. In Your Son's precious name I pray. Amen.

Guiding Light

My God, my Friend, what a relief it is to tell You my honest feelings. Right now I feel as though I'm living with a wicked giant, a giant not named Goliath, but cancer. He invaded my life and lurks in the deep crevices of my mind no matter what I'm doing or where I am. I tiptoe around him because at any minute he might awaken and threaten me. Will he devour me little by little or in one bite? This giant creates stress for my whole family as we wait for test results and struggle with life-and-death decisions. Lord, help me make it a priority, no matter how I feel or how busy I am, that I daily spend time with You in Your Word and in prayer. Every time I read a portion of Scripture, I grow deeper in my faith in You and more certain of Your love for me. You are my guiding light to slay cancer just as David slew Goliath. I praise You, Lord, for guiding me. And I thank You for encouraging me through stories of people like David. I can face this giant because You are with me! In Jesus' name I pray. Amen.

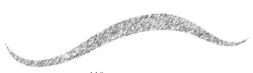

Impatience While Waiting

Heavenly Father, being still and waiting is not easy! I've been waiting five days for the results of my MRI and CT scan. I want answers now! Grant me an extra measure of patience, knowing Your timing is perfect! Shield me from Satan's attacks whenever I begin to doubt. Your Holy Word invites me to trust in You with *all* my heart, to lean not on my own understanding, and to acknowledge Your plans. Thank You, Lord, for never giving up on me as I struggle through this process. Merciful God, accept my prayer for the sake of Jesus. Amen.

Inevitable Death

O God, whose days are without end and whose mercies cannot be numbered, we implore You to make us deeply aware of the shortness and uncertainty of life. Let Your Holy Spirit lead us in faith, in holiness, and in righteousness all our days that, when we have served You in our generation we may be gathered unto our fathers, through Jesus Christ, our Lord. Amen. (LUTHERAN WORSHIP AGENDA, © 1984 Concordia Publishing House, pp. 370–71.)

Jars of Clay

Gracious Father, people often comment on my strength in coping with unremitting anxiety. This strength is not mine but Yours. "We have this treasure in jars of clay, to show that the surpassing power belongs to God and not to us. We are afflicted in every way, but not crushed; perplexed, but not driven to despair; persecuted, but not forsaken; struck down, but not destroyed" (2 Corinthians 4:7–9). You never promised me a stress-free life; in fact, Jesus said I would have tribulation. But You guarantee strength and hope from Your Spirit and from Your Sacraments. I rejoice that I can come to You as weary as I am, and You will always give me rest. Your Holy Supper will always sustain me. In Jesus' name. Amen.

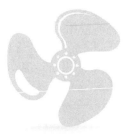

Lighten the Load

Almighty Creator, thank You for helping me find laughter in spite of what I've been through and all that lies ahead for me. Keep me from being so consumed with my health that I forget to enjoy Your gift of humor. I praise You for the powerful healing it brings to my heart, mind, and soul. The joy of Your presence is my strength. That joy is not based on temporary circumstances but is permanently rooted in my relationship with You. Let Your face smile on me and be gracious to me, and give me Your peace. Amen.

Loneliness

Precious Savior, at the cross You were deserted by Your closest disciples, and You endured the loneliness of being forsaken by Your Father. You know my loneliness. Comfort and strengthen me, I pray, with the knowledge of Your constant presence. Remind me that You will never leave me or forsake me. Help me to trust in You for every need and to learn to be content in every situation. Amen. (*PORTALS OF PRAYER*)

Peace in the Storms of Life

Lord Jesus, the stiller of storms,
the voice in the whirlwind, speak
to us Your words of peace and
focus our minds on You.
Give us strength, courage,
and wisdom to endure
the storms of life and to
see in You the peace that passes
all understanding, for You live
and reign with the Father
and the Holy Spirit, one God,
now and forever. Amen.

(*VISITATION*, p. 80)

Protection

Divine Lord, You showed Your love for me in Jesus, my Savior. Spread Your protecting wings over me. Uphold me amid suffering and pain. Give me strength to face the days with patience and the long nights with quieted nerves. Put my mind at ease as I remember Your love, which daily blots out all my sins. Keep me in Your grace. Each day give me a fuller measure of faith as I receive Your blessings through Jesus, my everlasting Friend. Amen. (*VISITATION*, p. 6)

Radiation Treatment

Merciful Lord, as I lie on the cold, narrow radiation table, my eyes are fixed on You, my Good Shepherd. You gather me into Your comforting arms and carry me close to Your heart. Although my tears flow through the tattooing procedure, a peacefulness encircles me from Your grace. Your rod and staff soothe the discomfort from radiation burns. Your sustaining hands give my worn-down body strength in my weakness. Thank You for Your Son, Jesus Christ, who guarantees me eternal life through His suffering and death. Amen.

Recurrence

Dear Lord Jesus, during the last years of being in remission, I've wondered whether a recurrence would be more difficult than the initial diagnosis. Now I know. Nothing that I've been through in the past, including this latest challenge, equaled the fear, anxiety, and confusion I felt on hearing that initial diagnosis. Yes, the familiarity of hearing that my cancer has recurred makes it feel easier, and knowing how procedures have advanced help to calm me. The friendly faces at the doctor's office and hospital bring comfort, yet I still experience major setbacks. I draw strength from Your Word: "May the God of hope fill you with all joy and peace in believing, so that by the power of the Holy Spirit you may abound in hope" (Romans 15:13). In Jesus' holy name. Amen.

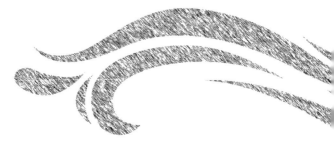

Rejoice Daily

Thank You, dear Father, through my Savior Jesus Christ, for teaching me daily to rejoice and be glad that I am Your child, that my sins are forgiven, and that I will live in heaven with You someday. I also rejoice that I am made in Your likeness and have a sense of humor. I'm learning that being able to laugh at movies, funny cards, and even at myself is a great stress relief. Give me wisdom to find pleasure in ordinary events, despite my brokenness, and to live life to the fullest. Jesus, my Savior, You are the source of my happiness and contentment. Guide me to focus on the fact that it is not the trials I have but what I do with them that makes the difference. "A joyful heart is good medicine, but a crushed spirit dries up the bones" (Proverbs 17:22). In Jesus' name. Amen.

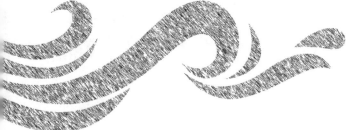

Repentance

Merciful Father, grant us Your divine aid, that we may not fall into temptation or be led in the way of destruction. Look not on our sins, nor on their account deny our prayer, but lead us into true repentance, that we may truly lament our sins and receive from the depth of Your mercy full pardon of all our transgressions; through the merit of Your Son, our Savior Jesus Christ. Amen. (*BLESSINGS*, p. 48)

Response to a Diagnosis

Heavenly Father, You have given the blessings of medicine and those who capably use it. For a treatable diagnosis, I thank You and pray for the success of future treatments. For a negative diagnosis, I thank You that I now know the cause of my misery. Give me strength to bear whatever comes my way, and if it is Your will, grant me recovery. Send me the Spirit, that I may entrust my body and soul into Your loving hands. For Jesus' sake I ask it. Amen. (*PORTALS OF PRAYER*)

Salvation

God, I want a real relationship with You. I admit that many times I've chosen to go my own way instead of Your way. Please forgive me my sins. Jesus, thank You for dying on the cross to pay the full penalty for all my sins. Show me my true value in Your eyes. Through Your love and Your power, make me the person You created me to be. In Your holy name I pray. Amen. (*BLESSINGS*, p. 48)

Spouse

Gracious Father, You have covered our marriage with Your grace as we have experienced the ups and downs in life. For this we praise You. It's challenging to have our routines now revolve around my cancer. Yet cancer has helped us clarify what we value. We give thanks for each new day, for helping us to ignore the little things that used to frustrate us and to pause to count how You bless us despite my affliction. Forgive me when I am short-tempered. Grant my spouse understanding. And help us to reflect that You are the head of our home and without You we are nothing. All glory, praise, and honor to You, our God and King. Amen.

Surgery: Before an Operation

Heavenly Father, be with me as I prepare for surgery. Take every fear out of my heart. Into Your hands I commend myself, trusting You for healing according to Your will. Grant my family peace, knowing I am in Your care. Give wisdom to the doctors and nurses, that all they do will bring about a speedy recovery. Forgive my sins. Comfort me with the assurance of my salvation through the precious blood of Your Son, Jesus Christ. O Lord of life and death, hear my prayer for Jesus' sake. Amen.

Surgery: After an Operation

Bless the Lord, O my soul, and all that is within me, bless His holy name. You have fulfilled Your promise to be with me during my surgery. When I was weak and helpless, You were my strength. Bless me with a restful day and refreshing sleep this night. Give me patience during my healing. O gracious Father, I cast all my cares on You, for I know that You care for me. Hear my prayer for the sake of Jesus Christ, my Savior. Amen. (Adapted from LUTHERAN BOOK OF PRAYER, © 1951 Concordia Publishing House, p. 156.)

You have been my constant
help and shield
as I have waited in hope.

Your steadfast love
never ceases;
Your mercies are new
each morning.

Surgery: Recovery

Lord Jesus, in this time of recovery from surgery, bring to me Your nurturing and healing presence, that my time of recovery may be quick and complete and I may return to my life whole and healed; for You live and reign with the Father and the Holy Spirit, now and forever. Amen. (*VISITATION*, p. 98)

Telling My Family

Lord Jesus Christ, I feel so inadequate for the task of telling my family and loved ones that I have cancer. I'm still having a problem accepting this myself. I plead for wisdom and direction because this is a delicate balancing act to be honest without scaring them and to talk at their comprehension level. Give them understanding when I can't attend their special events. Heal any rifts among us. Together, we need to be strong. Draw us all closer to one another, to You, and to our heavenly Father as we put our trust in You. Amen.

Thanksgiving

Gracious God, my prayers have been answered! Today I had excellent reports from my doctors, which mean no more appointments for a year! I rejoice and praise You for listening to my prayers. You have been my constant help and shield as I have waited in hope. In You, my heart rejoices. Forgive me for the times I questioned Your will for my life. Your steadfast love never ceases; Your mercies are new each morning. You are the Great Physician, my personal Good Shepherd, and my almighty Savior. Great is Your faithfulness! Amen.

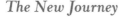

The New Journey

Faithful Shepherd, it's difficult adjusting to and accepting all the changes that happen with cancer. I used to get things done. Not now. Everything takes so much energy. Just doing the ordinary becomes extraordinary. I plead for fortitude and stamina. Stop me from pushing beyond healthy restraints. I praise You for the new perspective, for I have learned what is really important to me. I am filled with an unexplainable peace within, as my relationship with You has grown to a deeper level. I did not choose to have cancer, but You knew that all these things would mold me into a godlier person. I rest in Your grace. Amen.

Who's in Control?

Almighty Father, it is hard to surrender control to You or to anyone else. Keep me mindful that You are all knowing. You see the big picture of my life, while I see only this moment. Vulnerability engulfs me at each treatment and doctor's appointment. I don't like being told what to do and when. Help me accept that this reality is for my benefit. Although I cannot control what is happening to my body, I can control my attitude. I can make choices about resting and good nutrition. Yet while I get weary with all the decisions that I make, thank You, God, for making an eternal decision for me! I thank You that You chose me to be a recipient of Your salvation for the sake of Your Son's death and resurrection. I willingly surrender my life to Your control. Amen.

Why?

Heavenly Father, my humanness makes me search for answers to *Why me? Why now?* Although I may never know, You do. You know when I sit and rise up, what I am thinking and the words I will say. In love, You wove me together in my mother's womb. Knowing Your eyes are never off of me fills me with courage and contentment, even in the midst of cancer chaos. You will never forsake me. In faith I accept that Your plan for me is far greater than I can imagine. Help me approach this new chapter in life as a challenge, not a defeat. In Jesus' name. Amen.

Scripture
Verses

EXODUS 33:14

And He said, "My presence will go with you, and I will give you rest."

NUMBERS 6:24–26

The LORD bless you and keep you; the LORD make His face to shine upon you and be gracious to you; the LORD lift up His countenance upon you and give you peace.

DEUTERONOMY 31:6, 8

Be strong and courageous. Do not fear or be in dread of them, for it is the LORD your God who goes with you. He will not leave you or forsake you. . . . It is the LORD who goes before you. He will be with you; He will not leave you or forsake you. Do not fear or be dismayed.

JOSHUA 1:9

Have I not commanded you? Be strong and courageous. Do not be frightened, and do not be dismayed, for the LORD your God is with you wherever you go.

1 SAMUEL 16:7

But the LORD said to Samuel, "Do not look on his appearance or on the height of his stature, because I have rejected him. For the LORD sees not as man sees: man looks on the outward appearance, but the LORD looks on the heart."

NEHEMIAH 8:10

And do not be grieved, for the joy of the LORD is your strength.

JOB 11:18–19

And you will feel secure, because there is hope; you will look around and take your rest in security. You will lie down, and none will make you afraid;

PROVERBS 3:5–6

Trust in the LORD with all your heart, and do not lean on your own understanding. In all your ways acknowledge Him, and He will make straight your paths.

PROVERBS 17:22

A joyful heart is good medicine, but a crushed spirit dries up the bones.

ISAIAH 26:3–4

You keep him in perfect peace whose mind is stayed on You, because he trusts in You. Trust in the LORD forever for the LORD God is an everlasting rock.

ISAIAH 41:10

Fear not, for I am with you; be not dismayed, for I am your God; I will strengthen you, I will help you, I will uphold you with My righteous right hand.

ISAIAH 40:31

But they who wait for the LORD shall renew their strength; they shall mount up with wings like eagles; they shall run and not be weary; they shall walk and not faint.

JEREMIAH 17:7

Blessed is the man who trusts in the LORD, whose trust is the LORD.

JEREMIAH 29:11

For I know the plans I have for you, declares the LORD, plans for welfare and not for evil, to give you a future and a hope.

LAMENTATIONS 3:22–23

The steadfast love of the LORD never ceases; His mercies never come to an end; they are new every morning; great is Your faithfulness.

> Therefore do not be anxious about tomorrow, for tomorrow will be anxious for itself. Sufficient for the day is its own trouble.
>
> Matthew 6:34

MATTHEW 11:28–29

Come to Me, all who labor and are heavy laden, and I will give you rest. Take My yoke upon you, and learn from Me, for I am gentle and lowly in heart, and you will find rest for your souls.

LUKE 12:24–26

Consider the ravens: they neither sow nor reap, they have neither storehouse nor barn, and yet God feeds them. Of how much more value are you than the birds! And which of you by being anxious can add a single hour to his span of life? If then you are not able to do as small a thing as that, why are you anxious about the rest?

JOHN 3:16–17

For God so loved the world, that He gave His only Son, that whoever believes in Him should not perish but have eternal life. For God did not send His Son into the world to condemn the world, but in order that the world might be saved through Him.

Peace I leave with you;
  My peace I give to you.
Not as the world gives do
  I give to you. Let not
your hearts be troubled,
  neither let them be afraid.

John 14:27

JOHN 16:33

I have said these things to you, that in Me you may have peace. In the world you will have tribulation. But take heart; I have overcome the world.

ROMANS 5:1–5

Therefore, since we have been justified by faith, we have peace with God through our Lord Jesus Christ. Through Him we have also obtained access by faith into this grace in which we stand, and we rejoice in hope of the glory of God. More than that, we rejoice in our sufferings, knowing that suffering produces endurance, and endurance produces character, and character produces hope, and hope does not put us to shame, because God's love has been poured into our hearts through the Holy Spirit who has been given to us.

ROMANS 8:16–18

The Spirit Himself bears witness with our spirit that we are children of God, and if children, then heirs—heirs of God and fellow heirs with Christ, provided we suffer with Him in order that we may also be glorified with Him. For I consider that the sufferings of this present time are not worth comparing with the glory that is to be revealed to us.

ROMANS 8:26

Likewise the Spirit helps us in our weakness. For we do not know what to pray for as we ought, but the Spirit Himself intercedes for us with groanings too deep for words.

ROMANS 8:28

And we know that for those who love God all things work together for good, for those who are called according to His purpose.

For I am sure that neither death nor life, nor angels nor rulers, nor things present nor things to come, nor powers, nor height nor depth, nor anything else in all creation, will be able to separate us from the love of God in Christ Jesus our Lord.

Romans 8:38–39

ROMANS 10:17

So faith comes from hearing, and hearing through the word of Christ.

ROMANS 12:11–12

Do not be slothful in zeal, be fervent in spirit, serve the Lord. Rejoice in hope, be patient in tribulation, be constant in prayer.

ROMANS 15:13

May the God of hope fill you with all joy and peace in believing, so that by the power of the Holy Spirit you may abound in hope.

1 CORINTHIANS 10:13

No temptation has overtaken you that is not common to man. God is faithful, and He will not let you be tempted beyond your ability, but with the temptation He will also provide the way of escape, that you may be able to endure it.

2 CORINTHIANS 1:3–4

Blessed be the God and Father of our Lord Jesus Christ, the Father of mercies and God of all comfort, who comforts us in all our affliction, so that we may be able to comfort those who are in any affliction, with the comfort with which we ourselves are comforted by God.

2 CORINTHIANS 4:7–9

But we have this treasure in jars of clay, to show that the surpassing power belongs to God and not to us. We are afflicted in every way, but not crushed; perplexed, but not driven to despair; persecuted, but not forsaken; struck down, but not destroyed.

2 CORINTHIANS 4:16–18

So we do not lose heart. Though our outer self is wasting away, our inner self is being renewed day by day. For this light momentary affliction is preparing for us an eternal weight of glory beyond all comparison, as we look not to the things that are seen but to the things that are unseen. For the things that are seen are transient, but the things that are unseen are eternal.

2 CORINTHIANS 12:9

"My grace is sufficient for you, for My power is made perfect in weakness." Therefore I will boast all the more gladly of my weaknesses, so that the power of Christ may rest upon me.

Now to Him who is able to do far more abundantly than all that we ask or think, according to the power at work within us, to Him be glory in the church and in Christ Jesus throughout all generations, forever and ever. Amen.

Ephesians 3:20–21

PHILIPPIANS 4:6–7, 11

Do not be anxious about anything, but in everything by prayer and supplication with thanksgiving let your requests be made known to God.

And the peace of God, which surpasses all understanding, will guard your hearts and your minds in Christ Jesus. . . . Not that I am speaking of being in need, for I have learned in whatever situation I am to be content.

COLOSSIANS 2:6–7

Therefore, as you received Christ Jesus the Lord, so walk in Him, rooted and built up in Him and established in the faith, just as you were taught, abounding in thanksgiving.

TITUS 3:4–7

When the goodness and loving kindness of God our Savior appeared, He saved us, not because of works done by us in righteousness, but according to His own mercy, by the washing of regeneration and renewal of the Holy Spirit, whom He poured out on us richly through Jesus Christ our Savior, so that being justified by His grace we might become heirs according to the hope of eternal life.

HEBREWS 4:15–16

For we do not have a high priest who is unable to sympathize with our weaknesses, but one who in every respect has been tempted as we are, yet without sin. Let us then with confidence draw near to the throne of grace, that we may receive mercy and find grace to help in time of need.

> Now faith is the assurance of things hoped for, the conviction of things not seen.
>
> Hebrews 11:1

HEBREWS 12:1–2

Therefore, since we are surrounded by so great a cloud of witnesses, let us also lay aside every weight, and sin which clings so closely, and let us run with endurance the race that is set before us, looking to Jesus, the founder and perfecter of our faith, who for the joy that was set before Him endured the cross, despising the shame, and is seated at the right hand of the throne of God.

JAMES 1:2–5

Count it all joy, my brothers, when you meet trials of various kinds, for you know that the testing of your faith produces steadfastness. And let steadfastness have its full effect, that you may be perfect and complete, lacking in nothing. If any of you lacks wisdom, let him ask God, who gives generously to all without reproach, and it will be given him.

Blessed be the God and Father of our Lord Jesus Christ! According to His great mercy, He has caused us to be born again to a living hope through the resurrection of Jesus Christ from the dead.

1 Peter 1:3

1 PETER 3:15

In your hearts honor Christ the Lord as holy, always being prepared to make a defense to anyone who asks you for a reason for the hope that is in you; yet do it with gentleness and respect.

1 PETER 5:7

Casting all your anxieties on Him, because He cares for you.

1 PETER 5:10

And after you have suffered a little while, the God of all grace, who has called you to His eternal glory in Christ, will Himself restore, confirm, strengthen, and establish you.

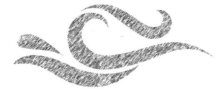

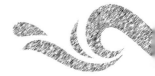

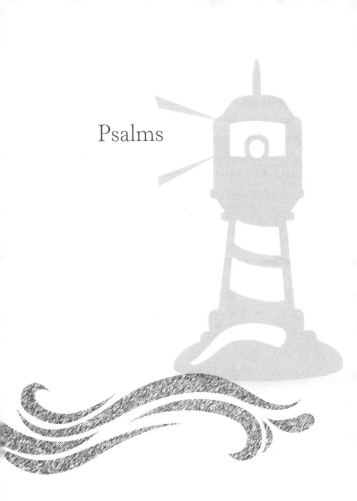

Psalms

Peace

PSALM 4:1, 3, 8

Answer me when I call, O God of my righteousness! You have given me relief when I was in distress. Be gracious to me and hear my prayer! . . . But know that the LORD has set apart the godly for Himself; the LORD hears when I call to Him. . . . In peace I will both lie down and sleep; for You alone, O LORD, make me dwell in safety.

Deliverance

PSALM 6:2–4, 6, 9

Be gracious to me, O LORD, for I am languishing; heal me, O LORD, for my bones are troubled. My soul also is greatly troubled. But You, O LORD—how long? Turn, O LORD, deliver my life; save me for the sake of Your steadfast love. . . . I am weary with my moaning; every night I flood my bed with tears; I drench my couch with my weeping. . . . The LORD has heard my plea; the LORD accepts my prayer.

Strength
PSALM 9:9–10

The LORD is a stronghold for the oppressed, a stronghold in times of trouble. And those who know Your name put their trust in You, for You, O LORD, have not forsaken those who seek You.

Assurance
PSALM 10:17

O LORD, You hear the desire of the afflicted; You will strengthen their heart; You will incline Your ear.

Strength
PSALM 18:1–3, 25, 28–30

I love You, O LORD, my strength. The LORD is my rock and my fortress and my deliverer, my God, my rock, in whom I take refuge, my shield, and the horn of my salvation, my stronghold. I call upon the LORD, who is worthy to be praised, and I am saved from my enemies. . . . With the merciful You show Yourself merciful; with the blameless man You show Yourself blameless. . . . For it is You who light my

145

lamp; the Lord my God lightens my darkness. For by You I can run against a troop, and by my God I can leap over a wall. This God—His way is perfect; the word of the Lord proves true; He is a shield for all those who take refuge in Him.

Trust

PSALM 23

The Lord is my shepherd; I shall not want. He makes me lie down in green pastures. He leads me beside still waters. He restores my soul. He leads me in paths of righteousness for His name's sake. Even though I walk through the valley of the shadow of death, I will fear no evil, for You are with me; Your rod and Your staff, they comfort me. You prepare a table before me in the presence of my enemies; You anoint my head with oil; my cup overflows. Surely goodness and mercy shall follow me all the days of my life, and I shall dwell in the house of the Lord forever.

Guidance

PSALM 25:1, 4–6, 10, 15–16, 18, 21

To You, O LORD, I lift up my soul. . . . Make me to know Your ways, O LORD; teach me Your paths. Lead me in Your truth and teach me, for You are the God of my salvation; for You I wait all the day long. Remember Your mercy, O LORD, and Your steadfast love, for they have been from of old. . . . All the paths of the LORD are steadfast love and faithfulness, for those who keep His covenant and His testimonies. . . . My eyes are ever toward the LORD, for He will pluck my feet out of the net. Turn to me and be gracious to me, for I am lonely and afflicted. . . . Consider my affliction and my trouble, and forgive all my sins. . . . May integrity and uprightness preserve me, for I wait for You.

Trust

PSALM 28:6–7

Blessed be the LORD! For He has heard the voice of my pleas for mercy. The LORD is my strength and my shield; in Him my heart trusts, and I am helped; my heart exults, and with my song I give thanks to Him.

Assurance
PSALM 30:5

Weeping may tarry for the night, but joy comes with the morning.

Mercy
PSALM 31:5, 9, 14, 24

Into Your hand I commit my spirit; You have redeemed me, O LORD, faithful God. . . . Be gracious to me, O LORD, for I am in distress; my eye is wasted from grief; my soul and my body also. . . . But I trust in You, O LORD; I say, "You are my God." . . . Be strong, and let your heart take courage, all you who wait for the LORD!

Hope/Trust
PSALM 33:18, 20–22

Behold, the eye of the LORD is on those who fear Him, on those who hope in His steadfast love. . . . Our soul waits for the LORD; He is our help and our shield. For our heart is glad in Him, because we trust in His holy name. Let Your steadfast love, O LORD, be upon us, even as we hope in You.

Deliverance
PSALM 34:4–5, 7–8, 15, 18–19

I sought the LORD, and He answered me and delivered me from all my fears. Those who look to Him are radiant, and their faces shall never be ashamed. . . . The angel of the LORD encamps around those who fear Him, and delivers them. Oh, taste and see that the LORD is good! Blessed is the man who takes refuge in Him! . . . The eyes of the LORD are toward the righteous and His ears toward their cry. . . . The LORD is near to the brokenhearted and saves the crushed in spirit. Many are the afflictions of the righteous, but the LORD delivers him out of them all.

Hope

PSALM 39:4–6, 7, 12

O LORD, make me know my end and what is the measure of my days; let me know how fleeting I am! Behold, You have made my days a few handbreadths, and my lifetime is as nothing before You. Surely all mankind stands as a mere breath!

Surely a man goes about as a shadow! Surely for nothing they are in turmoil; . . . And now, O Lord, for what do I wait? My hope is in You. . . . Hear my prayer, O LORD, and give ear to my cry; hold not Your peace at my tears!

Praise

PSALM 40:1, 5, 11

I waited patiently for the LORD; He inclined to me and heard my cry. . . . You have multiplied, O LORD my God, Your wondrous deeds and Your thoughts toward us; none can compare with You! I will proclaim and tell of them, yet they are more than can be told. . . . As for You, O LORD, You will not restrain Your mercy from me; Your steadfast love and Your faithfulness will ever preserve me!

Comfort

PSALM 42:5–8

Why are you cast down, O my soul, and why are you in turmoil within me? Hope in God; for I shall again praise Him, my salvation and my God. My soul is cast down within me; therefore I remember you from the land of Jordan and of Hermon, from Mount Mizar. Deep calls to deep at the roar of Your waterfalls; all Your breakers and Your waves have gone over me. By day the LORD commands His steadfast love, and at night His song is with me, a prayer to the God of my life.

Strength

PSALM 46:1–7, 10–11

God is our refuge and strength, a very present help in trouble. Therefore we will not fear though the earth gives way, though the mountains be moved into the heart of the sea, though its waters roar and foam, though the mountains tremble at its swelling. There is a river whose streams make glad the city of God, the holy habitation of the Most High. God is in the midst of her; she shall not be moved; God will help her when morning dawns. The nations rage, the kingdoms totter; He utters His voice, the earth melts. The LORD of hosts is with us; the God of Jacob is our fortress. . . . "Be still, and know that I am God. I will be exalted among the nations, I will be exalted in the earth!" The LORD of hosts is with us; the God of Jacob is our fortress.

Trust
PSALM 56:4

In God, whose word I praise, in God I trust; I shall not be afraid. What can flesh do to me?

Salvation
PSALM 62:1–2, 5–6, 8

For God alone my soul waits in silence; from Him comes my salvation. He only is my rock and my salvation, my fortress; I shall not be greatly shaken. . . . For God alone, O my soul, wait in silence, for my hope is from Him. He only is my rock and my salvation, my fortress; I shall not be shaken. . . . Trust in Him at all times, O people; pour out your heart before Him; God is a refuge for us.

Steadfast Love
PSALM 63:7–8

For You have been my help, and in the shadow of Your wings I will sing for joy. My soul clings to You; Your right hand upholds me.

Strength
PSALM 73:23–24, 26

Nevertheless, I am continually with You; You hold my right hand. You guide me with Your counsel, and afterward You will receive me to glory. . . . My flesh and my heart may fail, but God is the strength of my heart and my portion forever.

Refuge and Fortress
PSALM 91:1–2, 11

He who dwells in the shelter of the Most High will abide in the shadow of the Almighty. I will say to the LORD, "My refuge and my fortress, my God, in whom I trust." . . . For He will command His angels concerning you to guard you in all your ways.

Assurance
PSALM 94:19

When the cares of my heart are many, Your consolations cheer my soul.

Faithfulness
PSALM 105:4, 38–42

Seek the LORD and His strength; seek His presence continually! . . . Egypt was glad when they departed, for dread of them had fallen upon it. He spread a cloud for a covering, and fire to give light by night. They asked, and He brought quail, and gave them bread from heaven in abundance. He opened the rock, and water gushed out; it flowed through the desert like a river. For He remembered His holy promise, and Abraham, His servant.

Love

PSALM 116:1–7

I love the LORD, because He has heard my voice and my pleas for mercy. Because He inclined His ear to me, therefore I will call on Him as long as I live. The snares of death encompassed me; the pangs of Sheol laid hold on me; I suffered distress and anguish. Then I called on the name of the LORD: "O LORD, I pray, deliver my soul!" Gracious is the LORD, and righteous; our God is merciful. The LORD preserves the simple; when I was brought low, He saved me. Return, O my soul, to your rest; for the LORD has dealt bountifully with you.

Comfort

PSALM 119:49–50, 90, 105, 114

Remember Your word to Your servant, in which You have made me hope. This is my comfort in my affliction, that Your promise gives me life. . . . Your faithfulness endures to all generations; You have established the earth, and it stands fast. . . . Your word is a lamp to my feet and a light to my path. . . . You are my hiding place and my shield; I hope in Your word.

God's Faithfulness
PSALM 121:1–3, 5, 8

I lift up my eyes to the hills. From where does my help come? My help comes from the LORD, who made heaven and earth. He will not let your foot be moved; He who keeps you will not slumber. . . . The LORD is your keeper; the LORD is your shade on your right hand. . . . The LORD will keep your going out and your coming in from this time forth and forevermore.

Assurance
PSALM 126:5–6

Those who sow in tears shall reap with shouts of joy! He who goes out weeping, bearing the seed for sowing, shall come home with shouts of joy, bringing his sheaves with him.

Omnipotent God
PSALM 139:1–18

O LORD, You have searched me and known me! You know when I sit down and when I rise up; You discern my thoughts from afar. You search out my path and my lying down and are acquainted with all my ways. Even before a word is on my tongue, behold, O LORD, You know it altogether. You hem me in, behind and before, and lay Your hand upon me. Such knowledge is too wonderful for me; it is high; I cannot attain it. Where shall I go from Your Spirit? Or where shall I flee from Your presence? If I ascend to heaven, You are there! If I make my bed in Sheol, You are there! If I take the wings of the morning and dwell in the uttermost parts of the sea, even there Your hand shall lead me, and Your right hand shall hold me. If I say, "Surely the darkness shall cover me, and the light about me be night," even the darkness is not dark to You; the night is bright as the day, for darkness is as light with You. For You formed my inward parts; You knitted me together in my mother's womb. I praise You, for I am fearfully and wonderfully made. Wonderful are Your works; my soul knows it very well. My frame was not hidden from You, when I was being made in secret, intricately woven in the depths of the earth. Your eyes saw my unformed substance; in Your book were written, every one of them, the days that were formed for me, when as yet there was none of them. How precious to me are Your thoughts, O God! How vast is the sum of them! If I would count them, they are more than the sand. I awake, and I am still with You.

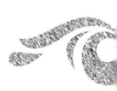

Hymns

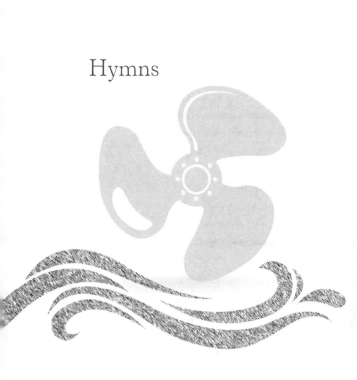

A Mighty Fortress Is Our God

A mighty fortress is our God,
A trusty shield and weapon;
He helps us free from ev'ry need
That hath us now o'ertaken.
The old evil foe
Now means deadly woe;
Deep guile and great might
Are his dread arms in fight;
On earth is not his equal.

With might of ours can naught be done,
Soon were our loss effected;
But for us fights the valiant One,
Whom God Himself elected.
Ask ye, Who is this?
Jesus Christ it is,
Of Sabaoth Lord,
And there's none other God;
He holds the field forever.

Though devils all the world should fill,
All eager to devour us,

We tremble not, we fear no ill;
They shall not overpow'r us.
This world's prince may still
Scowl fierce as he will,
He can harm us none.
He's judged; the deed is done;
One little word can fell him.

The Word they still shall let remain
Nor any thanks have for it;
He's by our side upon the plain
With His good gifts and Spirit.
And take they our life,
Goods, fame, child, and wife,
Though these all be gone,
Our vict'ry has been won;
The Kingdom ours remaineth.

Abide, O Dearest Jesus

Abide, O dearest Jesus,
Among us with Your grace
That Satan may not harm us
Nor we to sin give place.

Abide, O dear Redeemer,
Among us with Your Word,
And thus now and hereafter
True peace and joy afford.

Abide with heav'nly brightness
Among us, precious Light;
Your truth direct and keep us
From error's gloomy night.

Abide with richest blessings
Among us, bounteous Lord;
Let us in grace and wisdom
Grow daily through Your Word.

Abide with Your protection
Among us, Lord, our strength,
Lest world and Satan fell us
And overcome at length.

Abide, O faithful Savior,
Among us with Your love;
Grant steadfastness and help us
To reach our home above.

Amazing Grace

Amazing grace—how sweet the sound—
That saved a wretch like me!
I once was lost but now am found,
Was blind but now I see!

The Lord has promised good to me,
His Word my hope secures;
He will my shield and portion be
As long as life endures.

Through many dangers, toils, and snares
I have already come;
His grace has brought me safe thus far,
His grace will lead me home.

Yes, when this flesh and heart shall fail
And mortal life shall cease,
Amazing grace shall then prevail
In heaven's joy and peace.

When we've been there ten thousand years,
Bright shining as the sun,
We've no less days to sing God's praise
Than when we'd first begun.

Be Still, My Soul

Be still, my soul; the Lord is on your side;
Bear patiently the cross of grief or pain;
Leave to your God to order and provide;
In ev'ry change He faithful will remain.
Be still, my soul; your best, your heav'nly Friend
Through thorny ways leads to a joyful end.

Be still, my soul; your God will undertake
To guide the future as He has the past.
Your hope, your confidence let nothing shake;
All now mysterious shall be bright at last.

Be still, my soul; the waves and winds still know
His voice who ruled them while He dwelt below.

Be still, my soul; though dearest friends depart
And all is darkened in this vale of tears;
Then you will better know His love, His heart,
Who comes to soothe your sorrows and your fears.
Be still, my soul; your Jesus can repay
From His own fullness all He takes away.

Be still, my soul; the hour is hast'ning on
When we shall be forever with the Lord,
When disappointment, grief, and fear are gone,
Sorrow forgot, love's purest joys restored.
Be still, my soul; when change and tears are past,
All safe and blessèd we shall meet at last.

Come, My Soul, with Every Care

Come, my soul, with ev'ry care,
Jesus loves to answer prayer;
He Himself has bid thee pray,
Therefore will not turn away.

Thou art coming to a King,
Large petitions with thee bring;
For His grace and pow'r are such
None can ever ask too much.

With my burden I begin:
Lord, remove this load of sin;
Let Thy blood, for sinners spilt,
Set my conscience free from guilt.

Lord, Thy rest to me impart,
Take possession of my heart;
There Thy blood-bought right maintain
And without a rival reign.

While I am a pilgrim here,
Let Thy love my spirit cheer;
As my guide, my guard, my friend,
Lead me to my journey's end.

Show me what is mine to do;
Ev'ry hour my strength renew.
Let me live a life of faith;
Let me die Thy people's death.

Come unto Me, Ye Weary

"Come unto Me, ye weary,
And I will give you rest."
O blessèd voice of Jesus,
Which comes to hearts oppressed!
It tells of benediction,
Of pardon, grace, and peace,
Of joy that hath no ending,
Of love that cannot cease.

"Come unto Me, ye wand'rers,
And I will give you light."
O loving voice of Jesus,
Which comes to cheer the night!
Our hearts were filled with sadness,
And we had lost our way;
But Thou hast brought us gladness
And songs at break of day.

"Come unto Me, ye fainting,
And I will give you life."
O cheering voice of Jesus,
Which comes to aid our strife!
The foe is stern and eager,
The fight is fierce and long;

But Thou hast made us mighty
And stronger than the strong.

"And whosoever cometh,
I will not cast him out."
O patient love of Jesus,
Which drives away our doubt,
Which, though we be unworthy
Of love so great and free,
Invites us very sinners
To come, dear Lord, to Thee!

God Loved the World So
That He Gave

God loved the world so that He gave
His only Son the lost to save,
That all who would in Him believe
Should everlasting life receive.

Christ Jesus is the ground of faith,
Who was made flesh and suffered death;
All then who trust in Him alone
Are built on this chief cornerstone.

God would not have the sinner die;
His Son with saving grace is nigh;
His Spirit in the Word declares
How we in Christ are heaven's heirs.

Be of good cheer, for God's own Son
Forgives all sins which you have done;
And, justified by Jesus' blood,
Your Baptism grants the highest good.

If you are sick, if death is near,
This truth your troubled heart can cheer:
Christ Jesus saves your soul from death;
That is the firmest ground of faith.

Glory to God the Father, Son,
And Holy Spirit, Three in One!
To You, O blessèd Trinity,
Be praise now and eternally!

God Moves in a Mysterious Way

God moves in a mysterious way
His wonders to perform;
He plants His footsteps in the sea
And rides upon the storm.

Judge not the Lord by feeble sense,
But trust Him for His grace;
Behind a frowning providence
Faith sees a smiling face.

His purposes will ripen fast,
Unfolding ev'ry hour;
The bud may have a bitter taste,
But sweet will be the flow'r.

Blind unbelief is sure to err
And scan His work in vain;
God is His own interpreter,
And He will make it plain.

You fearful saints, fresh courage take;
The clouds you so much dread
Are big with mercy and will break
In blessings on your head.

Have No Fear, Little Flock

Have no fear, little flock;
Have no fear, little flock,
For the Father has chosen
To give you the Kingdom;
Have no fear, little flock!

Have good cheer, little flock;
Have good cheer, little flock,
For the Father will keep you
In His love forever;
Have good cheer, little flock!

Praise the Lord high above;
Praise the Lord high above,
For He stoops down to heal you,
Uplift and restore you;
Praise the Lord high above!

Thankful hearts raise to God;
Thankful hearts raise to God,
For He stays close beside you,
In all things works with you;
Thankful hearts raise to God!

How Sweet the Name of Jesus Sounds

How sweet the name of Jesus sounds
In a believer's ear!
It soothes our sorrows, heals our wounds,
And drives away our fear.

It makes the wounded spirit whole
And calms the heart's unrest;
'Tis manna to the hungry soul
And to the weary, rest.

Dear name! The rock on which I build,
My shield and hiding place;
My never-failing treasury filled
With boundless stores of grace.

O Jesus, shepherd, guardian, friend,
My Prophet, Priest, and King,
My Lord, my life, my way, my end,
Accept the praise I bring.

How weak the effort of my heart,
How cold my warmest thought!
But when I see Thee as Thou art,
I'll praise Thee as I ought.

Till then I would Thy love proclaim
With ev'ry fleeting breath;
And may the music of Thy name
Refresh my soul in death!

I Am Trusting Thee, Lord Jesus

I am trusting Thee, Lord Jesus,
Trusting only Thee;
Trusting Thee for full salvation,
Great and free.

I am trusting Thee for pardon;
At Thy feet I bow,
For Thy grace and tender mercy
Trusting now.

I am trusting Thee for cleansing
In the crimson flood;
Trusting Thee to make me holy
By Thy blood.
I am trusting Thee to guide me;

Thou alone shalt lead,
Ev'ry day and hour supplying
All my need.

I am trusting Thee for power;
Thine can never fail.
Words which Thou Thyself shalt give me
Must prevail.

I am trusting Thee, Lord Jesus;
Never let me fall.
I am trusting Thee forever
And for all.

If Thou But Trust in God
to Guide Thee

If thou but trust in God to guide thee
And hope in Him through all thy ways,
He'll give thee strength, whate'er betide thee,
And bear thee through the evil days.
Who trusts in God's unchanging love
Builds on the rock that naught can move.

What can these anxious cares avail thee,

These never-ceasing moans and sighs?
What can it help if thou bewail thee
O'er each dark moment as it flies?
Our cross and trials do but press
The heavier for our bitterness.

Be patient and await His leisure
In cheerful hope, with heart content
To take whate'er thy Father's pleasure
And His discerning love hath sent,
Nor doubt our inmost wants are known
To Him who chose us for His own.

God knows full well when times of gladness
Shall be the needful thing for thee.
When He has tried thy soul with sadness
And from all guile has found thee free,
He comes to thee all unaware
And makes thee own His loving care.

Nor think amid the fiery trial
That God hath cast thee off unheard,
That he whose hopes meet no denial
Must surely be of God preferred.
Time passes and much change doth bring
And sets a bound to ev'rything.
All are alike before the Highest;

'Tis easy for our God, we know,
To raise thee up, though low thou liest,
To make the rich man poor and low.
True wonders still by Him are wrought
Who setteth up and brings to naught.

Sing, pray, and keep His ways unswerving,
Perform thy duties faithfully,
And trust His Word; though undeserving,
Thou yet shalt find it true for thee.
God never yet forsook in need
The soul that trusted Him indeed.

In God, My Faithful God

In God, my faithful God,
I trust when dark my road;
Great woes may overtake me,
Yet He will not forsake me.
My troubles He can alter;
His hand lets nothing falter.

My sins fill me with care,
Yet I will not despair.

I build on Christ, who loves me;
From this rock nothing moves me.
To Him I will surrender,
To Him, my soul's defender.

If death my portion be,
It brings great gain to me;
It speeds my life's endeavor
To live with Christ forever.
He gives me joy in sorrow,
Come death now or tomorrow.

O Jesus Christ, my Lord,
So meek in deed and word,
You suffered death to save us
Because Your love would have us
Be heirs of heav'nly gladness
When ends this life of sadness.

"So be it," then, I say
With all my heart each day.
Dear Lord, we all adore You,
We sing for joy before You.
Guide us while here we wander
Until we praise You yonder.

Jesus Christ Is Risen Today

Jesus Christ is ris'n today, Alleluia!
Our triumphant holy day, Alleluia!
Who did once upon the cross, Alleluia!
Suffer to redeem our loss. Alleluia!

Hymns of praise then let us sing, Alleluia!
Unto Christ, our heav'nly king, Alleluia!
Who endured the cross and grave, Alleluia!
Sinners to redeem and save. Alleluia!

But the pains which He endured, Alleluia!
Our salvation have procured; Alleluia!
Now above the sky He's king, Alleluia!
Where the angels ever sing. Alleluia!

Sing we to our God above, Alleluia!
Praise eternal as His love; Alleluia!
Praise Him, all ye heav'nly host, Alleluia!
Father, Son, and Holy Ghost. Alleluia!

Jesus Loves Me

Jesus loves me! This I know,
For the Bible tells me so.
Little ones to Him belong;
They are weak, but He is strong.

Refrain: Yes, Jesus loves me!
           Yes, Jesus loves me!
           Yes, Jesus loves me!
           The Bible tells me so.

Jesus loves me! He who died
Heaven's gates to open wide.
He has washed away my sin,
Lets His little child come in. *Refrain*

Just as I Am, without One Plea

Just as I am, without one plea
But that Thy blood was shed for me
And that Thou bidd'st me come to Thee,
O Lamb of God, I come, I come.

Just as I am and waiting not
To rid my soul of one dark blot,
To Thee, whose blood can cleanse each spot,
O Lamb of God, I come, I come.

Just as I am, though tossed about
With many a conflict, many a doubt,
Fightings and fears within, without,
O Lamb of God, I come, I come.

Just as I am, poor, wretched, blind;
Sight, riches, healing of the mind,
Yea, all I need, in Thee to find,
O Lamb of God, I come, I come.

Just as I am, Thou wilt receive,
Wilt welcome, pardon, cleanse, relieve;
Because Thy promise I believe,
O Lamb of God, I come, I come.

Just as I am; Thy love unknown
Has broken ev'ry barrier down;
Now to be Thine, yea, Thine alone,
O Lamb of God, I come, I come.

Let Us Ever Walk with Jesus

Let us ever walk with Jesus,
Follow His example pure,
Through a world that would deceive us
And to sin our spirits lure.
Onward in His footsteps treading,
Pilgrims here, our home above,
Full of faith and hope and love,
Let us do the Father's bidding.
Faithful Lord, with me abide;
I shall follow where You guide.

Let us suffer here with Jesus
And with patience bear our cross.
Joy will follow all our sadness;
Where He is, there is no loss.
Though today we sow no laughter,
We shall reap celestial joy;
All discomforts that annoy
Shall give way to mirth hereafter.
Jesus, here I share Your woe;
Help me there Your joy to know.

Let us also live with Jesus.
He has risen from the dead
That to life we may awaken.
Jesus, You are now our head.
We are Your own living members;
Where You live, there we shall be
In Your presence constantly,
Living there with You forever.
Jesus, let me faithful be,
Life eternal grant to me.

My Hope Is Built on Nothing Less

My hope is built on nothing less
Than Jesus' blood and righteousness;
No merit of my own I claim
But wholly lean on Jesus' name.

Refrain: On Christ, the solid rock, I stand;
All other ground is sinking sand.

When darkness veils His lovely face,
I rest on His unchanging grace;

In ev'ry high and stormy gale
My anchor holds within the veil. *Refrain*

His oath, His covenant and blood
Support me in the raging flood;
When ev'ry earthly prop gives way,
He then is all my hope and stay. *Refrain*

When He shall come with trumpet sound,
Oh, may I then in Him be found,
Clothed in His righteousness alone,
Redeemed to stand before His throne! *Refrain*

The Lord's My Shepherd, I'll Not Want

The Lord's my shepherd, I'll not want;
He makes me down to lie
In pastures green; He leadeth me
The quiet waters by.

My soul He doth restore again
And me to walk doth make
Within the paths of righteousness,
E'en for His own name's sake.

Yea, though I walk in death's dark vale,
Yet will I fear no ill;
For Thou art with me, and Thy rod
And staff me comfort still.

My table Thou hast furnished
In presence of my foes;
My head Thou dost with oil anoint,
And my cup overflows.

Goodness and mercy all my life
Shall surely follow me;
And in God's house forevermore
My dwelling place shall be.

The Will of God Is Always Best

The will of God is always best
And shall be done forever;
And they who trust in Him are blest;
He will forsake them never.
He helps indeed
In time of need;

He chastens with forbearing.
They who depend
On God, their friend,
Shall not be left despairing.

God is my comfort and my trust,
My hope and life abiding;
And to His counsel, wise and just,
I yield, in Him confiding.
The very hairs,
His Word declares,
Upon my head He numbers.
By night and day
God is my stay;
He never sleeps nor slumbers.

Lord, this I ask, O hear my plea,
Deny me not this favor:
When Satan sorely troubles me,
Then do not let me waver.
O guard me well,
My fear dispel,
Fulfill Your faithful saying:
All who believe
By grace receive
An answer to their praying.

When life's brief course on earth is run
And I this world am leaving,
Grant me to say, "Your will be done,"
Your faithful Word believing.
My dearest Friend,
I now commend
My soul into Your keeping;
From sin and hell,
And death as well,
By You the vict'ry reaping.

Savior, like a Shepherd Lead Us

Savior, like a shepherd lead us;
Much we need Your tender care.
In Your pleasant pastures feed us,
For our use Your fold prepare.
Blessèd Jesus, blessèd Jesus,
You have bought us; we are Yours.
Blessèd Jesus, blessèd Jesus,
You have bought us; we are Yours.

We are Yours; in love befriend us,
Be the guardian of our way;
Keep Your flock, from sin defend us,
Seek us when we go astray.
Blessèd Jesus, blessèd Jesus,
Hear us children when we pray.
Blessèd Jesus, blessèd Jesus,
Hear us children when we pray.

You have promised to receive us,
Poor and sinful though we be;
You have mercy to relieve us,
Grace to cleanse, and pow'r to free.
Blessèd Jesus, blessèd Jesus,
Early let us turn to You.
Blessèd Jesus, blessèd Jesus,
Early let us turn to You.

Early let us seek Your favor,
Early let us do Your will;
Blessèd Lord and only Savior,
With Your love our spirits fill.
Blessèd Jesus, blessèd Jesus,
You have loved us, love us still.
Blessèd Jesus, blessèd Jesus,
You have loved us, love us still.

What a Friend We Have in Jesus

What a friend we have in Jesus,
All our sins and griefs to bear!
What a privilege to carry
Ev'rything to God in prayer!
Oh, what peace we often forfeit;
Oh, what needless pain we bear—
All because we do not carry
Ev'rything to God in prayer!

Have we trials and temptations?
Is there trouble anywhere?
We should never be discouraged—
Take it to the Lord in prayer.
Can we find a friend so faithful
Who will all our sorrows share?
Jesus knows our ev'ry weakness—
Take it to the Lord in prayer.

Are we weak and heavy laden,
Cumbered with a load of care?
Precious Savior, still our refuge—
Take it to the Lord in prayer.
Do thy friends despise, forsake thee?
Take it to the Lord in prayer.
In His arms He'll take and shield thee;
Thou wilt find a solace there.

When Peace, like a River

When peace, like a river, attendeth my way;
When sorrows, like sea billows, roll;
Whatever my lot, Thou hast taught me to say,
It is well, it is well with my soul.

Refrain:
It is well (It is well)
with my soul, (with my soul),
It is well, it is well with my soul.

Though Satan should buffet,
though trials should come,

Let this blest assurance control,
That Christ hath regarded my helpless estate
And hath shed His own blood for my soul.
Refrain

He lives—oh, the bliss of this glorious thought;
My sin, not in part, but the whole,
Is nailed to His cross, and I bear it no more.
Praise the Lord, praise the Lord, O my soul!
Refrain

And, Lord, haste the day
when our faith shall be sight,
The clouds be rolled back as a scroll,
The trumpet shall sound
and the Lord shall descend;
Even so it is well with my soul.
Refrain